The Fertility Awareness

A guide for all those who want a greater understanding of
natural family planning methods

In the same series

The Fertility Awareness Workbook

The Complete Guide to Natural Family Planning for the Woman Who
Wants to Conceive, and the Woman Who Doesn't

by

Barbara Kass-Annese & Dr Hal Danzer

THORSONS PUBLISHING GROUP
Wellingborough · New York

First UK Edition 1986

Kass-Annese, Barbara
The Fertility awareness workbook.
1. Natural family planning
I. Title   II. Danzer, Hal C.
613.9'434   RG136.5

ISBN 0-7225-1272-4

Printed and bound in Great Britain

ACKNOWLEDGEMENTS

The authors express their thanks to:

Susan Alcott
John Altamura
Bart Andrews
Joe Bectol
Peter Bersin
Dana Chalberg
Blake Conway
Gareth Esersky
William Grace
Michelle Martino
H. Roy Matlen
F. Clyde Petersen
Tom Rachels
Kiran Rana
Sherri Robb
Barbara S. Rollins

who made THE FERTILITY AWARENESS WORKBOOK

and its predecessor, PATTERNS, possible.

CONTENTS

Although this book has been prepared by experts in the field of fertility awareness, it does not purport to take the place of qualified medical advice and treatment when appropriate. Please contact your doctor and/or a fertility awareness instructor regarding medical matters and problems related to natural family planning and fertility awareness methods.

INTRODUCTION

Are there times when you have been mystified by your own body and reproductive organs and feel that you should have been told more?

Did you know that a woman can become pregnant only during a few days of each menstrual cycle?

Did you know that a woman can become pregnant on Friday from having intercourse on Monday?

Did you know that having intercourse during menstrual bleeding can sometimes lead to pregnancy?

Do you want a safe and effective alternative to the pill, intrauterine device, spermicide, condom, diaphragm and rhythm methods of birth control?

Did you know there are natural ways that are safe and effective in avoiding pregnancy that can also be an aid for achieving pregnancy?

If you use a diaphragm, spermicide or condom, would you like to know why you do not have to use your method of birth control each time you have intercourse?

Do you feel it's time to know more — to no longer be mystified about your body and reproduction?

THE FERTILITY AWARENESS WORK-BOOK will answer all of these questions and more.

This workbook has been written for those who want a greater understanding of their bodies. *It is not only a book about avoiding and achieving pregnancy, but also a book for those who want to learn what is normal and healthy for them.*

THE FERTILITY AWARENESS WORK-BOOK will explain and illustrate the most up-to-date information about women's and men's reproductive systems. It focuses on the naturally occurring changes that take place within a woman's body. *These changes, called FERTILITY SIGNS, can be used to determine the days during each menstrual cycle when a woman can and cannot become pregnant.*

Knowledge about fertility signs has existed for some time but has not been widely available until now. This book was designed to provide you with this knowledge — knowledge that can be used in many rewarding ways throughout your lifetime.

All of nature is made of patterns — as a woven fabric is made of patterns of threads, one overlapping the other, creating an intricate tapestry.

The seasons represent patterns of nature, each

leading slowly and fittingly into the next.

Our bodies, like the seasons, also have patterns. Our youth slips inevitably into adolescence, into adulthood, then into middle-age and finally into the latter years. During this life-cycle our bodies reveal various patterns to us.

The set of patterns that we concentrate on in this book — the patterns of fertility — can be thought of as a special language of the woman's body.

THE FERTILITY AWARENESS WORKBOOK will show you how to understand this language.

This workbook provides you with accurate information about reproduction. It also includes revealing information about a woman's body and provides specific instruction on the use of two methods of family planning:
  natural family planning and the
  fertility awareness method.

This book has a clear logic to it. It begins with a brief history of natural family planning, followed by basic chapters on how the reproductive systems of both women and men work. If you are to understand the body's language about fertility, then you should first learn exactly why the reproductive organs work the way they do. All of this basic knowledge is meant to help you increase your awareness of the normal and natural changes of the reproductive cycle.

Following the chapters on basics, there is a detailed explanation and description of the body's special language — fertility signs.

Knowing exactly what fertility signs are and how they work, as well as why they work, will give you confidence with your own personal method of family planning.

Next comes a section of step-by-step instructions on how to observe and record your fertility signs and how to prevent or achieve a pregnancy.

Because some couples experience difficulty achieving a pregnancy, infertility is also discussed.

Since any method of family planning has both advantages and disadvantages, this workbook closes with a discussion of these aspects as they concern natural family planning and fertility awareness methods.

As you begin reading about the facts of fertility awareness and end with considering your own feelings, we hope you find this awareness and information rewarding and enriching.

CHAPTER I

NATURAL FAMILY PLANNING AND FERTILITY AWARENESS METHODS
What Are They?

Almost everywhere you turn, you see and hear references to the word *natural* — natural food, natural childbirth and natural "lifestyles."

We also want to use the word *natural* in this original meaning — that which occurs in nature, like the natural workings of the human body. So when we say that you have natural information, we mean that your body actually does offer the signs we talk about, signs that are based on accurate, specific and available natural body language. They are called *fertility signs*.

Body Signs = Fertility Signs

Fertility signs let you know when you can get pregnant and when you cannot get pregnant. Proper use of these signs will let you know your *fertile days* —those days during the month when it is possible to become pregnant. Since you are able to know your fertile days, you can also know those days during the month when you cannot become pregnant. These days are known as *infertile days*.

Natural family planning (NFP) is a way of family planning that does not include the use of artificial birth control. Therefore, during fertile days, if you do not want to get pregnant, you do not have sexual intercourse.

On the other hand, if you do want to achieve pregnancy, then having intercourse during these fertile days offers the very highest possibility — the maximum chance — to become pregnant.

Fertility awareness method (FAM) is a family planning method also. Both NFP and FAM use the same naturally occurring fertility signs to guide you. However, with FAM you have a choice during your fertile days: if you do not choose to abstain from sexual intercourse, you can use a cervical cap, a diaphragm, a condom and/or a spermicide.

In other words, FAM teaches you how to identify those few days during each menstrual cycle when some form of contraception needs to be used so that pregnancy will not occur. This choice of what to do during the fertile days is the major difference between natural family planning and fertility awareness methods.

Regardless of the method used, the significant point is this: your body reveals fertility signs that enable you to identify the fertile and infertile days during each menstrual cycle and all of this is based on a natural language that is spoken by your body.

By learning this language, you can join the thousands of women and men who are now enjoying these alternative approaches to family planning!

CHAPTER II

A BIT OF HISTORY

Since the beginning of recorded history the desire for reliable methods to avoid pregnancy and enhance fertility has existed. Women beyond the healthy childbearing years or women who were ill were not expected to bear children. The woman who experienced repeated stillbirths or very difficult deliveries often sought to avoid future pregnancies. Times of war, famine or inability to adequately provide for the health and safety of a child were also important factors in the choice to delay pregnancy. As you can see by these examples, people throughout the ages had many of the same reasons for pregnancy avoidance as we do today.

How have people attempted to avoid pregnancy?

Beginning with pre-biblical times, people have used celibacy, breastfeeding, withdrawal, magical potions, charms and herbal mixtures — all to avoid pregnancy.

During the time of the ancient Hebrews one method used was a spongy substance placed inside the vagina to block sperm. Greek and Roman literature tells us of many methods of birth control, including tying up asparagus to be worn as a charm and vaginal suppositories made from honey and peppermint juice.

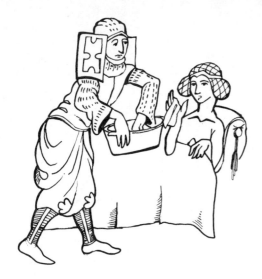

During the Middle Ages in Europe and Islam a number of recipes, many magical, were used to avoid pregnancy. One unusual recipe instructed a woman who did not want to become pregnant to soak a piece of cloth in the oil of a barberry tree and place it on the left side of her forehead. Another method suggested eating beans on an empty stomach and rubbing tar on the penis prior to intercourse as forms of birth control. A Moroccan ritual made use of a ring containing a special stone set in gold or silver. The man wore this ring during intercourse. If pregnancy was to be avoided, he would turn the ring so that the stone faced one of his fingers. In North Africa some tribal women ate a piece of honeycomb mixed with a few dead bees and placed between pieces of bread. Some Sumatran women placed a small ball of opium inside their vaginas.

A folk belief of Southern Russian women described taking a few drops of their menstrual blood and letting it flow into a hole made in the first egg of a young hen. The woman would bury the egg near a table in the room. The egg was left buried for 9 days and nights. When it was removed, the worms found in it were counted. It was believed that the number of worms represented the number of children the woman would have. If she threw the egg into fire, she wouldn't have children. If she desired children, she would throw the egg into water.

Other methods of birth control included douching solutions made of lemon juice and the husks of mahogany nuts, algae or seaweed placed inside the vagina before intercourse, carrying a child's tooth, and drinking thyme and lavender tea.

Since fertility was usually not understood, it was often considered mystical. Slowly, as a truer understanding about the facts of physiology and reproduction became known, science and technology began to replace the magical.

Around the middle of the 18th century, although potions and ceremonies continued to be used, modern mechanical forms of birth control began emerging. The condom was one of the first of these to be introduced.

The birth control movement in America had begun by 1828. It included withdrawal, a vaginal sponge made from sheep's wool or silk, and douching solutions made from white oak bark, green tea, or vinegar and water. Although the use of the diaphragm emerged in Holland during the early 1880's, it was not introduced to American women until the early 1920's. Between the 1920's and 1930's the rhythm method, Grafenburg intrauterine silver ring and spermicides began to be used. From that point on several types of intrauterine devices were developed. And "the pill" entered the mainstream of American life during the 1960's.

Where does NFP fit into all of this? What kind of history does it have?

We know historically that in various areas throughout the world women have used and continue to use breastfeeding as a natural means of child spacing. Yet, compared to the thousands of real and "magical" methods of contraception that have evolved and been recorded, little has been written about other forms of natural family planning. There is limited information available about African and American Indian tribes, as well as other groups, who appear to have had some knowledge of their fertility cycles. It is known that these tribes did use one of the major fertility signs, cervical mucus, as a means to achieve or avoid pregnancy. It is still used by them today.

Over 150 years ago a researcher, Dr. Bischoff, found eggs present in the uterus and fallopian tubes of a female dog while the dog was bleeding — "in heat." Because of this discovery he assumed that women must also have eggs present during their menstrual bleeding. Therefore, he believed that women became pregnant if they had intercourse during their periods. As a result of his findings, a natural birth control schedule was developed. It stated that if pregnancy was to be avoided, intercourse should not occur during the menstrual period, as well as 5 days before it and 9 days after it.[1] It was considered that these were the days when the woman could become pregnant. We now know that just the opposite is true!

This "natural birth control" continued to be practiced until the 1930's, and countless women became pregnant trying to use this totally incorrect information.

However, not all past information was incorrect. As early as 1857, there were descriptions of women who believed they could tell when they were ovulating because once a month they experienced internal aching or a painful feeling in the area of the ovaries. (Ovulation is the release of the egg from the ovary.)

This pain with ovulation continued to be discussed and written about for years. In 1935, Dr. Cyrus Anderson wrote a paper entitled, "Teaching the Patient to Observe Symptoms of Ovulation." This paper discussed ovulation pain and how women could be taught to recognize it.[2]

Ovulation pain, as you will soon learn, can be used by some women as a fertility sign. One of the other fertility signs you will learn about is the temperature of the body at rest, known as basal body temperature. It was studied as early as 1876 by Dr. Marie Putnam Jacobi.[3] She found that the basal body temperature rises from low temperatures to higher temperatures at some point during the menstrual cycle.

Cervical mucus, another fertility sign, was also written about in the 1800's. In fact, around the mid-1800's it was observed that this mucus changed in amount and quality throughout the menstrual cycle. From these observations, it was believed that a particular kind of mucus was needed to achieve a pregnancy.

Finally, in 1929, the rhythm method was developed when two men, on opposite sides of the world and independent of each other, discovered that an egg is released from the ovary approximately 14 days before the next menstrual flow begins. This discovery formed the basis of the Ogina-Knaus Calendar Rhythm Method. This method is named after the two discoverers, Dr. Ogina and Dr. Knaus.

However, the rhythm method did not prove to be accurate enough to be used by all women as a form of birth control. This is because the success of the rhythm method is dependent upon a woman experiencing consistently regular cycles, an uncommon event for many. The life span of the egg and sperm were not then known, which also contributed to the ineffectiveness of the rhythm method.

In 1962, Dr. Hartman found that sperm could live in the woman's body for three days, while the egg lives for one day. This added up to a 4-day period of time during the menstrual cycle when a woman could become pregnant. We now know that if the proper conditions are present in the woman's body, sperm can live and remain capable of fertilizing the egg for a period of up to 5 days.

During the 1960's, an Australian team of physicians, Drs. John and Evelyn Billings, conducted extensive research of the cervical mucus. They were attempting to find a method of natural family planning that would be more accurate than the rhythm method. Consequently, their research led to the development of the Billings Method, also known as the cervical mucus method or ovulation method. This method is based on using the observations of the cervical mucus to determine the fertile and infertile days of the menstrual cycle.

Even before the development of the Billings Method, the sympto-thermal method of natural family planning was made available. This method is based on the use of the cervical mucus, basal body temperature and other symptoms of ovulation to determine the days of infertility and fertility.

All this adds up to the fact that reliable methods of natural family planning, the ovulation and sympto-thermal methods, have been used by people throughout the world for over 30 years!

How effective are these methods of natural family planning?

Before answering this question, it is important to acknowledge that a woman's and man's feelings about pregnancy play a very important part in how a method of birth control is used. Women and men who are motivated to avoid a pregnancy tend to use a method more carefully, and careful use means fewer pregnancies.

Because of this fact and others, effectiveness rates, or how successful a method of birth control is, are discussed in two ways. One is the theoretical effectiveness rate. This type of effectiveness rate tells us how well a method works when used perfectly. In other words, no mistakes are made on the parts of the clinician or instructor providing the birth control method or the person using the method. The second type of effectiveness rate is called use effectiveness. This is the real effectiveness of the method, taking into account human error made by the user of the method, the clinician or the instructor.

For example, if a couple using NFP did not abstain during a fertile time and the woman became pregnant, this would be called a user failure. A user failure may also be because of the inability of the couple to understand the method, and this may be due to the teacher, the couple or a combination of both.

If a couple using NFP perfectly becomes pregnant, this is a theoretical failure, a failure of the method to prevent pregnancy.

A 3-year study, supported by the Department

of Health, Education and Welfare and completed in 1979 at Cedar-Sinai Medical Center in Los Angeles, compared the effectiveness of ovulation method and the sympto-thermal method. Over 1200 couples participated in this study. It was found that the ovulation method was approximately 78% effective. This means that 22 out of every 100 women who began use of the method, and who did not stop using it for any reason, became pregnant within one year. The symptothermal method was determined to be approximately 89% use effective, which means that out of every 100 women who began use of this method and did not stop using it for any reason, 11 became pregnant within one year. The results of this particular study are generally similar to many others which have been conducted throughout the world.

Many of the pregnancies in this study occurred because people "took chances" and had intercourse during the fertile time, did not understand the use of the methods, or did not follow other instructions necessary for the effective use of these two methods.

The reason why the couples using the symptothermal (S-T) method experienced a lower number of pregnancies is not completely understood. However, the Cedar-Sinai Study and others, in addition to our own experience in working with these methods, suggest that for many people the S-T method is easier to teach, to learn and to use properly. The findings of this particular study, in addition to many others, have consistently suggested that the theoretical effectiveness rates of both methods are approximately equal. When instructed correctly by the teachers, in combination with the couples' understanding and proper use of the methods, the effectiveness rates are approximately 98%.

The effectiveness rates of the natural family planning methods are comparable with almost all of the other methods of contraception.[4]

	Theoretical Effectiveness	Use Effectiveness
Birth Control Pills	99.66%	90-94%
Condom and Spermicide	99+ %	95%
Intrauterine Device	97-99%	95%
Condom	97%	90%
Diaphragm	97%	83%
Spermicidal Foam	97%	78%

The fertility awareness method has an even briefer history than natural family planning.

About 5 years ago, groups of professionals active in family planning felt it to be important that women and men have complete information about their fertility patterns, regardless of whether or not they chose to use NFP.

Not only did they feel this information itself could enable people to avoid pregnancy naturally, but they also felt that it could be used in combination with other methods such as the diaphragm, spermicide and condoms.[*] Combining fertility sign information and other methods became known as Fertility Awareness Method (FAM). FAM provides people with the means to determine the few days during each menstrual cycle when they are fertile and another method of birth control is needed.

[*]See the Bibliography if you are interested in learning more about various methods of contraception.

Although to date there are FAM studies in progress, none have been completed documenting the effectiveness of the use of barrier and spermicidal methods of contraception during the fertile time. Many family planning professionals believe that the effectiveness rates should be about the same as the rates achieved when the diaphragm, condom and spermicide are used throughout the menstrual cycle.

Because FAM uses these other methods only during the fertile time, people may actually use them more conscientiously and correctly, resulting in fewer unplanned pregnancies.

The reasons why people choose to use natural family planning or fertility awareness method are certainly varied and complex. To some, NFP is a way of life. It is not only a method of birth control, but a total way that a woman and man relate to each other, spiritually, emotionally, and physically. NFP is a method that is compatible with particular teachings of various religions. For others, NFP is used because it is in keeping with their beliefs about their health. Some people desire to eliminate as many chemicals as possible from their lifestyle. And for some, natural family planning is the only method of birth control they can or want to use, due to prior physical and/or emotional problems with other methods of birth control. The numbers of people using the fertility awareness method appear to be growing because it seems that they wish to use the natural language of the body in combination with a method of birth control they are already comfortable using. In the end, the method chosen will depend upon a number of factors including the physical, emotional, sexual and spiritual needs of the person.

Now that we've briefly introduced natural family planning and fertility awareness methods to you, and given you an idea of how poorly reproduction was understood in the past, it's time to begin learning how well reproduction and these new methods of natural family planning are understood today.

[1]H. Arthur Allbutt, *Wife's Handbook* (4th ed.; London: Forder, 1887).

[2]Carl Gottfried Hartman, *Science and the Safe Period; a Compendium of Human Reproduction* (Baltimore: Williams and Wilkins, 1962).

[3]Ibid.

[4]Robert A. Hatcher, M.D., et al., *Contraceptive Technology* (New York: Irvington Publishers, 1979).

CHAPTER III

ALL THE PARTS *DOWN THERE* AND HOW THEY WORK
The Man

Men's and women's reproductive systems have similarities and obvious differences, and each goes through its own special and wondrous patterns to allow pregnancy to occur — at least some of the time.

Learning how these patterns and systems work and using the knowledge of fertility signs offer a couple choices about their love-making.

The **pituitary gland** is a small gland located in the base of the brain. Basically, it controls the reproductive system by sending hormonal signals in both men and women. (*Hormones* are chemicals that take messages from glands to other parts of the body, causing them to perform special and specific tasks.)

The pituitary gland begins to work more actively around the time a boy reaches the age of 8 to 12. This time of change, known as **puberty**, lasts about 4 years. During these years the major male hormone, **testosterone**, plays an important part in the development of the boy's body. For example, testosterone causes the growth of body hair and sex organs, including the penis. Sexual feelings also begin to increase under the influence of testosterone. This is the time a boy begins to experience "wet dreams," known as nocturnal emissions — a normal involuntary ejaculation which occurs when the boy is asleep. (Ejaculation is the release of semen from the penis.)

During puberty, the pituitary gland sends a

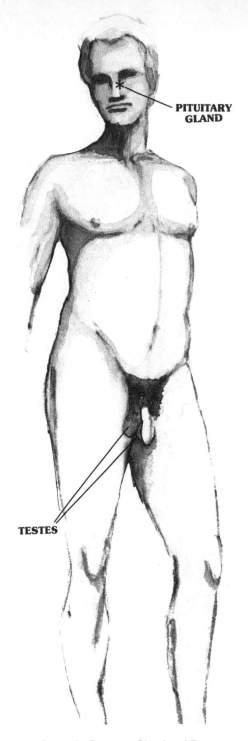

PITUITARY GLAND

TESTES

Figure 1—Pituitary Gland and Testes

message to the **testes**, the male sex glands.

The testes begin to produce sperm and testosterone. The testes are a pair of oval-shaped organs that produce about 50,000,000 sperm each day. They are protected by two sacs of loose, thin tissue known as the **scrotum**. The scrotum and testes are located on the outside of the man's body for a very specific reason. Their anatomical positioning keeps them cooler than normal body temperature. Cool temperature is needed for sperm production. Once sperm are produced in the testes, they travel to the **epididymis**, an area where they become fully developed. This is where they will wait until they begin their journey through the rest of the man's reproductive system.

When a man experiences sexual feelings, the sperm leave the epididymis and move along the **vas deferens**, a pair of 20-inch-long tubes that carry sperm to the **seminal vesicles**. These sac-like structures produce seminal fluid that nourishes the sperm. Sperm and seminal fluid continue traveling through the vas deferens, around the side of the bladder, to the **prostate gland**. This gland, the size and shape of an acorn, produces a thin, milky fluid which also nourishes the sperm. Sperm mixed with fluid from the seminal vesicles and prostate gland is called semen. Semen then moves into the passageway of the **ejaculatory duct**. During this entire process, the man's penis, a muscular organ, has become swollen. The swelling is caused by an increase in the amount of blood flowing into the tissues of the penis. A small tube that runs through the center of the penis is called the **urethra**. Usually the urethra serves as the exit for urine from the man's body. But, during ejaculation, the urethra serves as an exit for the semen. A pair of sac-like glands known as the **Cowpers**

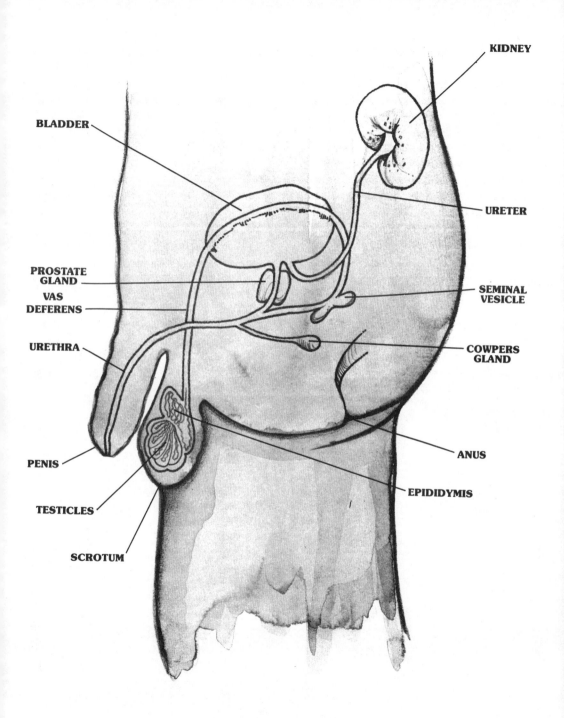

KIDNEY

BLADDER

URETER

PROSTATE
GLAND

VAS
DEFERENS

SEMINAL
VESICLE

URETHRA

COWPERS
GLAND

ANUS

PENIS

EPIDIDYMIS

TESTICLES

SCROTUM

Figure 2—Male Reproductive System

glands produce a fluid that also helps sperm live. When a man is sexually aroused and before he ejaculates, the fluid travels through the urethra to the tip of the penis.

Some researchers feel that these drops of fluid from the Cowpers glands contain enough sperm to cause a pregnancy. This means that if the tip of the penis touches the outside of the vagina during a woman's fertile time, pregnancy may occur. When the penis touches the vagina, it is called "genital to genital contact." As we will discuss later, *no genital to genital contact* should occur during the woman's fertile days if the couple wishes to avoid a pregnancy. When ejaculation is about to occur, the muscles in the penis and other parts of the reproductive system begin to contract or move. These muscle contractions are called orgasm, and they push the semen through the urethra to the outside of the man's body.

Two important facts to remember: the man is fertile every day from puberty until about the age of 70, and pregnancy can occur, if even just the tip of the penis touches the outside of the vagina.

CHAPTER IV

ALL THE PARTS *DOWN THERE* AND HOW THEY WORK
The Woman

The woman's fertility pattern is quite different from the man's. While the man is fertile every day, the woman is fertile approximately 5 to 7 days during each menstrual cycle. To understand why this is so is to learn how the woman's reproductive system works. This can be done by first looking at the part of the system located on the outside of the woman's body. This part is called the external genitalia.

At the top of the external genitalia is the **mons veneris** (named after Venus, the goddess of love). It is a pad of fatty tissue that covers the pubic bone and at puberty becomes covered with pubic hair. The mons veneris helps to protect the internal reproductive organs. Below it is the **vaginal opening**, a 3-inch to 4-inch-wide entrance leading into the **vaginal canal** and having a variety of functions. It allows for the final exit of menstrual blood from the body. The vaginal canal widens to allow for intercourse and also expands to aid in the birth of a baby. Often, at birth, a baby girl has a paper-thin tissue that partially and sometimes totally covers the vaginal opening. This tissue, known as the **hymen**, can be easily stretched by insertion of a tampon, finger or penis. Once this stretching occurs, irregular-looking pieces of the hymen are left around the vaginal opening. These pieces are known as the **hymenal tags.**

Located on either side of the vaginal opening are two sets of vaginal lips. The outer set is made of fatty tissue covered with skin that contains oil-producing glands. These outer lips are covered, to some degree, with pubic hair. The inner set of lips are hairless and do not contain oil-producing glands. This set is made of folds of soft skin. Together, the **labia majora** (outer lips) and **labia minora** (inner lips) protect the vaginal opening when a woman is not sexually aroused. When a woman does become sexually aroused, blood flows into the vaginal lips, causing them to fill with blood and flatten out away from the vagina — allowing for the insertion of the penis. The **clitoris**, a small pea-sized organ located below the mons veneris and above the vaginal opening, is made of the same kind of tissue as the penis. The clitoris becomes filled with blood during sexual arousal, causing it to become firm and erect. It contains many nerve endings which make it the main area of sexual arousal for many women. The clitoris is protected by a covering called the **hood**, which is formed by the joining of the inner lips above the clitoris.

Below the clitoris, and above the vaginal entrance, is the urinary opening called the **urethral meatus**. This opening is the entrance to the urethra, a tube leading to the bladder. The urinary opening serves as the passageway for the urine to travel from the bladder to the outside of the body. Below the vaginal opening is the **perineum**. This area of tissue is often cut during the birth of a baby when it is necessary to allow the baby easy passage out of the vaginal opening. The perineum also separates the vaginal opening from the **anus**, the muscular opening of the **rectum** that serves as the exit for the body's solid waste materials.

The **vulva** is the name given to all of the external genitalia that we've just described. Women often wonder if their vulva looks normal. The amount of pubic hair, size of the vaginal lips and clitoris form a unique "style" for each woman. If a woman places a mirror between her thighs, she can see her external sex organs. The woman comfortable doing this can become better acquainted with her body. She can learn what is normal for her. In other words, a woman who takes the time to look and touch these various parts of her body can learn to feel comfortable with her own body and gain a fuller understanding and awareness of it. This may help her overcome any shame and embarrassment about the outside of her reproductive system.

As we have mentioned, many of the external parts of the woman's reproductive system help to protect the internal reproductive organs. The internal reproductive organs work together to enable a woman to become pregnant and nourish the pregnancy through 9 months of development.

Beginning with the **uterus**, we see a hollow, muscular organ that is somewhat pear-shaped. It is only about 3 inches long and provides the space for the fetus to be nourished during the 9 months of development. The innermost lining of the uterus is called the **endometrium**. This lining becomes rich in blood supply and nutrients necessary for a pregnancy to occur and develop.

If the woman doesn't become pregnant during her cycle, the lining breaks down causing bleeding. This is called **menstruation**.

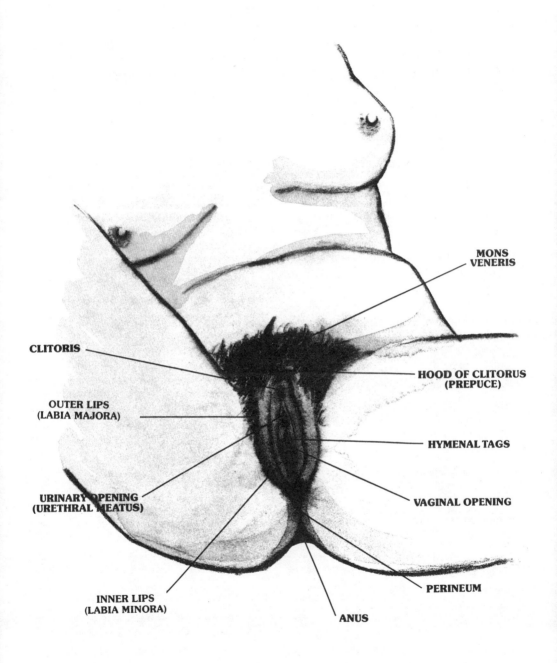

MONS
VENERIS

CLITORIS

HOOD OF CLITORUS
(PREPUCE)

OUTER LIPS
(LABIA MAJORA)

HYMENAL TAGS

URINARY OPENING
(URETHRAL MEATUS)

VAGINAL OPENING

INNER LIPS
(LABIA MINORA)

PERINEUM

ANUS

Figure 3—External Female Reproductive Anatomy

The menstrual blood leaves the uterus through its bottom part, known as the **cervix**. The cervix is often referred to as the neck of the uterus because it looks like a small neck sticking out at the very top of the vagina. The cervix has an opening that allows the sperm to enter the uterus during the fertile days of her menstrual cycle. The cervix also has glands made up of special cells that produce a fluid called **cervical mucus.** During the fertile days of the menstrual cycle, this mucus has a special consistency that allows sperm to live and travel through the woman's reproductive system to enable pregnancy to occur.

A 4-inch to 6-inch elastic, muscular tube is the connection between the vaginal opening and the cervix. Commonly called the birth canal or vaginal canal, this tube has the ability to expand during sexual arousal, allowing sexual intercourse. It also expands to allow the birth of a baby. When a woman is sexually aroused, the blood vessels in the lining of the vaginal canal become full, causing a slippery liquid to be produced. This liquid lubricates the vaginal canal, enabling a woman to have comfortable intercourse.

Vaginal and uterine muscles, as well as muscles around and in the reproductive organs, contract if a woman has experienced enough pleasure during lovemaking to have an orgasm.[*]

The primary sex organs, known as the **ovaries**, are located on each side of the uterus. Each ovary is about the size and shape of an almond. At birth, a baby girl has all of the immature eggs (called **ova**) in her ovaries that she will ever need. They number in the thousands and each is surrounded by a capsule called the **follicle**. The human egg can be compared to the chicken egg in a general way. The center of the chicken egg has a yolk surrounded by a white fluid and a shell to protect the whole egg. The human egg, smaller than a grain of sand, forms the center, with follicular fluid around it. All of this is surrounded by the follicle. At some point during each menstrual cycle an egg will fully develop and be released from its follicle and ovary. The egg is then picked up by one of the **fallopian** tubes. The fallopian tubes are a pair of narrow, muscular passageways. They are thin, about 4 inches in length and have finger-like ends called **fimbriae**. The fimbriae encircle the ovary and pick up the egg. The outer portion of the tube is where the egg will wait for only 12 to 24 hours. If sperm have not traveled through the uterus and up the fallopian tube before the time the egg has arrived, or within the next 24 hours, the egg will be absorbed by the body. It does not leave the body in the menstrual blood. If the egg is fertilized, it will begin a journey of approximately one week down the fallopian tube, into the uterus and burrow itself into the rich lining of the uterus, which has been preparing for the possibility of pregnancy. This is called **implantation**. The uterus lining is a perfect home for the fertilized egg, allowing it to develop into a baby within nine months.

For most young girls puberty begins between ages 8 and 13. As with the boy, the process lasts for about 4 years, allowing for physical and sexual maturity to take place. Generally, the first sign of puberty is breast development, followed by growth of underarm and pubic hair. One of the last events of puberty is the onset of a menstrual period, called the **menarche**. Although the menarche means the ovaries have reached an adult level of development, the release of the first egg may not begin for one to two years after this first menstrual period. Yet, once the eggs

[*]See the Bibliography for references if you want more detailed information about the changes in men's and women's bodies during lovemaking and orgasm.

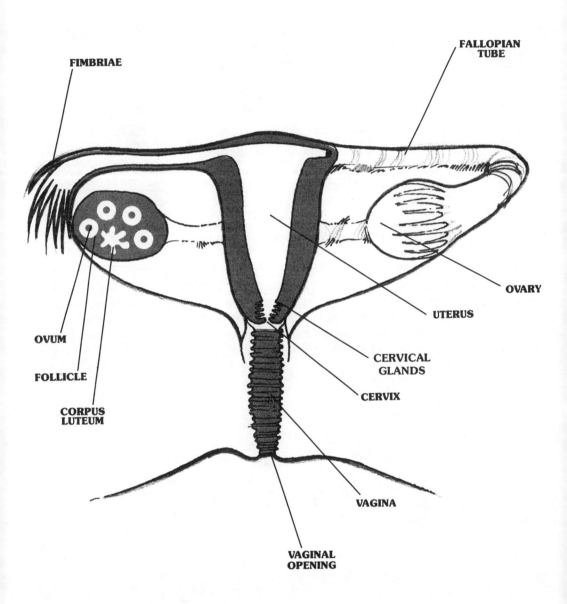

FIMBRIAE

FALLOPIAN
TUBE

OVARY

UTERUS

OVUM

CERVICAL
GLANDS

FOLLICLE

CERVIX

CORPUS
LUTEUM

VAGINA

VAGINAL
OPENING

Figure 4—Female Internal Reproductive Organs

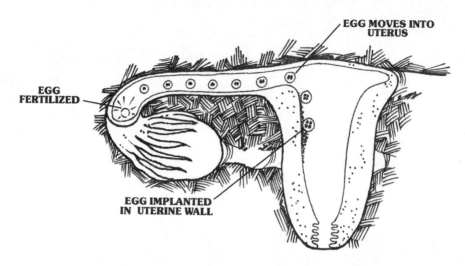

EGG MOVES INTO UTERUS

EGG FERTILIZED

EGG IMPLANTED IN UTERINE WALL

Figure 5—Fertilization and Implantation

begin to be released, the young girl is fertile and can become pregnant.

Usually the girl will release one egg during each fertility cycle — releasing approximately 400 eggs during her lifetime. This process is called **ovulation**.

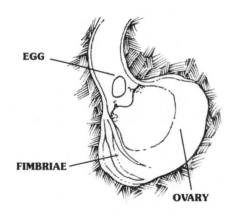

EGG

FIMBRIAE

OVARY

Figure 6—Ovulation

Ovulation is the MAIN EVENT of the fertility

cycle. The fertility cycle, commonly known as the **menstrual cycle**, spans many days, ranging from 22 to 35 days in length. It is not unusual for a woman's menstrual cycle to vary from 2 to 7 days in length from month to month. For example, the same woman may have cycles that are 25 days long, 27 days long, and still other cycles 32 days long. And that's okay — normal for her. It's also normal for the number of days and amount of bleeding to change with different menstrual cycles.

A menstrual cycle always begins the first day any sign of menstrual bleeding appears and ends the day before the next cycle of menstrual bleeding begins again. For example, Mary's menstrual bleeding began April 1. Her next menstrual bleeding began April 30. Therefore, her menstrual cycle during April was 29 days long.

About the time menstrual bleeding begins, the **pituitary gland** sends messages to the ovaries signaling them to begin their growth of eggs. The follicle and egg begin to grow. The

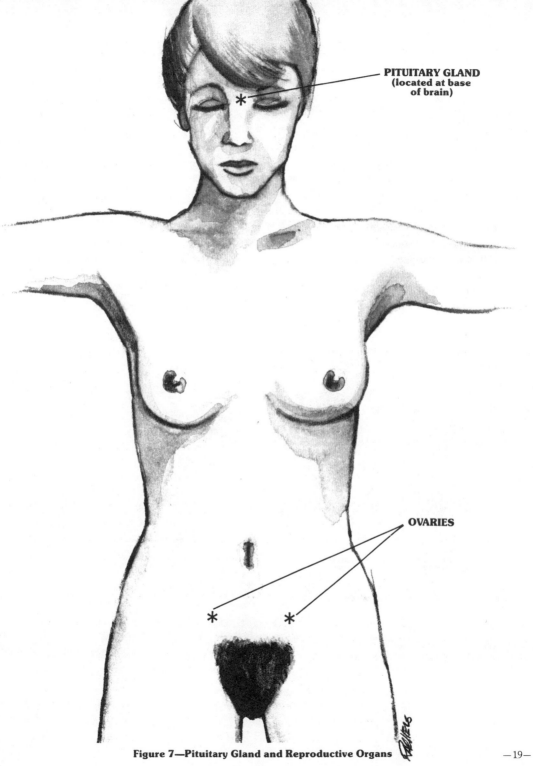

PITUITARY GLAND
(located at base
of brain)

OVARIES

Figure 7—Pituitary Gland and Reproductive Organs

—19—

follicle surrounding the egg also starts to produce one of the major female hormones, **estrogen**. The hormone estrogen is responsible for causing the young girl's body to develop into the body of a woman. Estrogen also causes the lining of the uterus to grow and develop the proper blood supply and nutrients necessary for implantation of the fertilized egg. A woman cannot feel this change. However, other changes caused by estrogen can be seen and felt; one is cervical mucus. **Fertile cervical mucus** is produced under the control of estrogen. Fertile mucus has certain qualities that will enable sperm to stay healthy and able to fertilize an egg for from three to five days. That means a woman can have intercourse on Monday and, if fertile mucus is present, the sperm can be waiting in the reproductive system to fertilize an egg — even if it isn't released from the ovary until Friday!

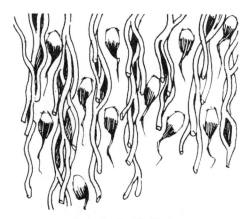

Figure 8—Fertile Mucus

The fact that sperm can live for up to 5 days is important to remember for the successful use of natural family planning. This cervical mucus may help filter out unhealthy sperm. It contains channels that form "super highways" that vibrate, helping to push the sperm up into the uterus.

Estrogen produces a slight rising of the uterus, causing the cervix to move into a higher position in the vaginal canal. Estrogen also causes the cervix to soften and its opening to widen. All of these changes help sperm to travel easily into the uterus. The changes in both mucus and the cervix can be observed by the woman, enabling her to determine her days of fertility. *Cervical mucus and changes in the cervix are two main fertility signs used to prevent or achieve a pregnancy.*

Once the egg has matured and estrogen is at a proper level in the woman's body, the pituitary gland sends another message to the ovary signaling the egg to be released. The egg leaves its follicle and enters the fallopian tube. Once this occurs, the follicle turns into an entirely different structure, now yellow in color. This is the **Corpus Luteum** (Latin for "yellow body"). The corpus luteum continues to produce estrogen though in smaller amounts. Now, it produces large amounts of **progesterone** — the second major female hormone. Once ovulation has taken place, progesterone controls the remainder of the menstrual cycle. One of its jobs is to change the lining of the uterus so that within 5 to 7 days after the egg has been released, the uterine lining is completely prepared. This preparation is necessary for implantation of a fertilized egg. Progesterone stops the ovaries from releasing more eggs, meaning once ovulation occurs, it will not happen again later in that same menstrual cycle. Occasionally a second egg will be released, but if that happens it will be within 24 hours after the release of the first egg. This explains the reason for non-identical, fraternal, twins. About one percent of all babies born are non-identical twins.

After one or perhaps two eggs are released, no more will be released during the cycle. Since there are no more eggs released, there is no further chance of pregnancy. This is another important factor in using fertility signs to prevent pregnancy.

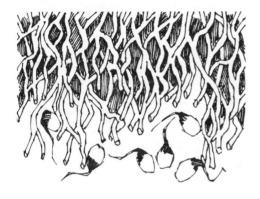

Figure 9—Infertile Mucus

Progesterone also causes the production of **infertile cervical mucus**. After ovulation the mucus produced destroys sperm and blocks it from traveling into the uterus. The cervix lowers in the vaginal canal and becomes firm, and the opening closes. These natural occurrences prevent sperm or any other foreign matter from entering the uterus and harming a pregnancy should one have occurred. Once again, these special changes in the mucus and cervix can enable a woman to identify the days when she is infertile, or not able to become pregnant.

In addition to changes in mucus and the cervix, changes in basal body temperature provide an invaluable sign to help a woman determine when she is no longer fertile. Body temperature rises significantly following ovulation compared to what it was before ovulation. It rises from about 3/10 (three-tenths or .3) of a degree to 1 full degree higher than the body temperature before ovul-

ation. This happens because progesterone is a heat-producing hormone. Once the temperature has risen, it will remain high for 12 to 16 days, or until the next menstrual cycle begins. This is because the corpus luteum produces progesterone and estrogen for about 12 to 16 days, keeping the uterine lining prepared for the possibility of pregnancy. If pregnancy doesn't occur, the corpus luteum stops working and the hormone levels decrease. Thus, the hormones are no longer present in the quantity needed to keep the uterine lining in place. The lining breaks down, accompanied by bleeding. This is the menstrual flow, which begins a new menstrual cycle. Menstrual cycles continue until the ovaries have "run out" of eggs. This takes place about the age of 45. Once bleeding has ceased for one full year, a woman has entered the menopause, and she can no longer become pregnant.

Menstrual bleeding is called MENSES from the Latin word for "monthly bleeding." It is more commonly referred to by a variety of names and phrases such as: "period," "friend," "curse," "falling off the roof," and "on the rag." Throughout history and even today, menstrual bleeding is often thought of as something "bad." There are many reasons for this. During ancient times bleeding was associated with the life process. This meant that life went on as long as the blood stayed in the body. To bleed meant to be injured and frequently to die. Therefore, for a woman to bleed and not be hurt was an unexplained mystery. Almost every religion and culture has written about this mystery of women, and often in a negative way. It was felt that women were possessed either by evil or by good spirits. For a period of time women were considered to be gods.

They were felt to possess supernatural powers. If women could control the life force, they could also control the weather, the growth of crops, birth and death.

This powerful godlike role given to women soon turned into a role very much the opposite. As soon as the early civilizations realized women who continued menstruating were not helping to increase the population, menstruation became a "curse." Women were said to be possessed by the devil and were called witches. When they were menstruating, they were considered to be dangerous to men. In fact, women were blamed for just about everything. If crops died, milk curdled, meat spoiled, or a tornado or hurricane came along, guess who was blamed? In fact, in some areas of the world, women had to live in special places away from their homes during menstruation. This was to protect everyone from harm since the look from a menstruating woman was said to soften men's bones and prevent them from fighting well during a battle.

Obviously this attitude about ·menstruation was based upon ignorance and carried a bit too far. Many women today still feel the effects of this history. Many women and men feel that menstruation is unclean, instead of viewing it as the end of one fertility cycle and the beginning of the next. Nothing more, nothing less.

TO REVIEW:

During the first part of the menstrual cycle, estrogen is the main female hormone. While the egg develops in its follicle, the follicle produces estrogen. Estrogen causes the cervix to rise, soften, open and produce fertile mucus. These changes let sperm live and travel to the egg. They can also help a woman identify the time when she can become pregnant.

Once the egg leaves its follicle, the follicle becomes the corpus luteum. The corpus luteum produces progesterone which causes the cervix to close and become plugged with infertile mucus. These changes help to protect a pregnancy if it should occur. The basal body temperature also rises. All of these changes help a woman identify the time when she cannot become pregnant.

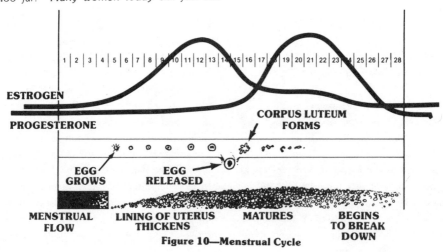

Figure 10—Menstrual Cycle

CHAPTER V

THE THREE MAJOR ONES
Primary Fertility Signs

In the spring a good gardener knows the signs for the time to plant. The pattern of the seasons is nature's language to the gardener. Nature's language to the woman is fertility signs.

You need to learn all you can about your fertility cycle so that sensible and intelligent choices can be made about your family planning. **Awareness is important.** In this section we emphasize a special kind of awareness — **fertility awareness** — learning about fertility signs and their patterns.

The 3 most important fertility signs are:

* **cervical mucus changes**
* **basal body temperature changes**
* **cervical changes**

Cervical Mucus

Cervical mucus is a substance that every woman produces naturally. It is one of the 3 most important fertility signs your body offers you and can be thought of as a special signal from your body, telling you about your reproductive system. It is a signal telling you when you are able to become pregnant, as well as when you are not able to become pregnant. Cervical mucus is normal; it is healthy; it is important and it can be easy to learn and understand its pattern.

This mucus is produced by very small glands in the cervix and it changes in ways that you can see and feel throughout your menstrual cycle. During certain days of the menstrual cycle, the mucus will be of either the fertile or infertile type. Fertile mucus is present during the time of ovulation when pregnancy can occur. Infertile mucus is present at other times of the menstrual cycle when pregnancy cannot occur. Remember! Fertile mucus helps a woman become pregnant. Infertile mucus helps prevent a woman from becoming pregnant.

Both fertile and infertile mucus have their own special:
> color
> amount
> feel

and you can learn to identify each kind.

After the menstrual flow ends, one of three changes will occur in the mucus pattern.

Change Number One: You may not have any mucus for one day or more. Days without any mucus are called "dry days." In fact, you may "feel dry" on the outside of your vagina. Some women notice this dryness toward the end of their menstrual flow because, in removing a tampon, they experience discomfort. Dryness may also be felt during love-making.

You may not experience the same amount of vaginal wetness while making love on these dry days as you experience at other times in your menstrual cycle.

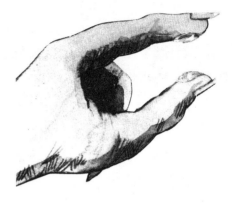

Figure 12—Creamy Mucus

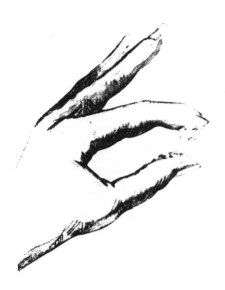

Figure 11—Pasty Mucus

Change Number Two: When the menstrual flow ends, you may produce a mucus that is sticky, pasty or crumbly. It sometimes resembles old-fashioned library paste, looking whitish-yellow on underwear. It is not a wet-feeling mucus. Since it has very little moisture, it causes the area around the vaginal opening to feel dry.

Change Number Three: When the menstrual flow ends, you may produce a wet-feeling mucus that appears creamy and white. This type of mucus may create a wet feeling around the vaginal opening.

In summary, once the menstrual flow ends, you may experience:

1. *A dry feeling at the opening of the vagina with no mucus present.*
2. *A dry feeling at the opening of the vagina with sticky, pasty, crumbly mucus.*
3. *A wet feeling at the opening of the vagina with a wet-feeling mucus.*

Regardless of whether you are dry or you begin to produce pasty or wet mucus after the menstrual flow ends, the closer the approach of ovulation, the wetter the mucus becomes.

This is due to the fact that in the beginning of the menstrual cycle, your body's estrogen level is low. As ovulation approaches, the increase of estrogen causes glands in the cervix to produce the wetter mucus.

In addition, the amount of mucus can increase, and it usually becomes clearer in color. It may even be pink, tinged with blood. It can be stretched between two fingers. This type of mucus has the appearance and texture of raw egg white. Known as Spinnbarkeit (pronounced Spin-bar-kite), German for "spider web," it can look like shimmering strands of a spider web. It is likely that you will notice a wet feeling at the opening of your vagina along with an increase of wet mucus on your underwear. Some women have misunderstood this wet mucus. They considered it to be the sign of a vaginal infection. This is not so!

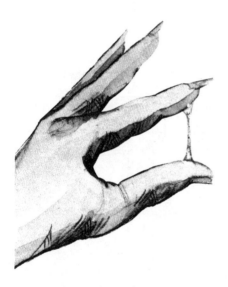

Figure 13—Stretchy Mucus

During the time when your mucus is the wettest and most slippery, your estrogen level is at its highest. This sign allows you to know that ovulation has taken place or will occur within a few days.

Soon after ovulation progesterone levels begin to rise in your body, causing other changes in the cervical mucus. As they rise, the mucus begins to lose its wet feeling. The wet feeling at the outside of your vaginal opening disappears, and the mucus becomes sticky, pasty and dry. Some women have a constant dry feeling at the outside of the vagina because they do not have any mucus for the remainder of their menstrual cycle. Other women continue to have the pasty type and dry vaginal sensation until their next menstrual cycle begins. A few days prior to menstrual bleeding some women notice a wet mucus and wet feeling at the outside of the vaginal opening. Though the mucus feels wet, it is not fertile mucus. It is merely a normal change for some women.

Many women notice these normal mucus changes throughout their menstrual cycles — the wet and dry feelings, the increase and decrease in vaginal secretions and the color changes — yet have never associated these changes with their normal fertility patterns.

Cervical mucus is the main fertility sign used to give advance notice that ovulation is going to happen.

Is it correct to say that ovulation took place on the day of the greatest amount of stretchy, wet mucus? NO! This type of mucus simply tells you that the time of ovulation is close.

We know that when menstrual bleeding ends. the appearance of any mucus, whether it is of the non-wet or wet quality, means an egg has begun growing and may soon be released.
WARNING!
The change from the non-wet, infertile type of mucus to the wet, fertile type of mucus can be difficult to see and feel. You may also miss detecting a small amount of fertile

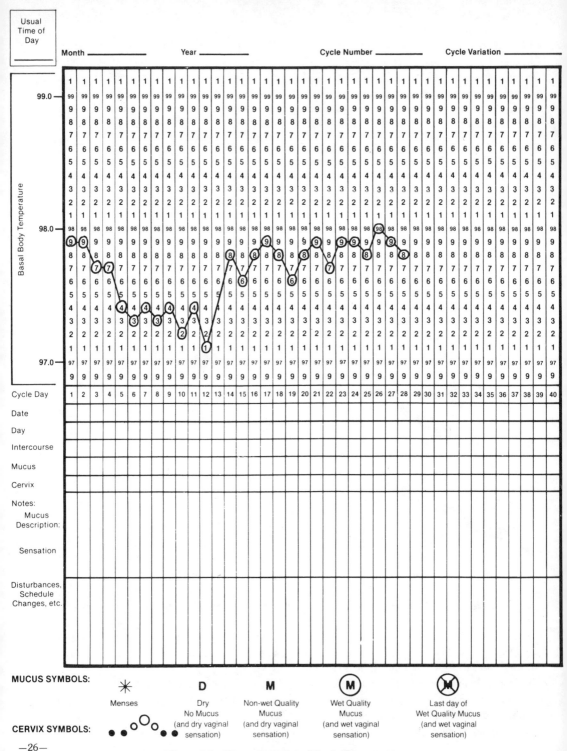

Figure 14—Changes in Basal Body Temperature

mucus mixed with infertile mucus. Therefore, after the menstrual bleeding ends, *any type of mucus that appears before ovulation is fertile.*

Basal Body Temperature

The second primary fertility sign is your basal body temperature. This is the temperature of your body at rest. When it is taken daily, you will see it rise and lower in a definite pattern that can. be used to aid in determining your fertile and infertile times. Remember, following ovulation the heat-producing hormone progesterone is produced by the corpus luteum. This causes your temperature to rise. You can use this temperature pattern in combination with your mucus changes to prevent or to achieve pregnancy.

When the menstrual flow begins, your temperature may still be high from the progesterone produced in your previous menstrual cycle. If it is, by the time the menstrual flow ends, your basal body temperature will have dropped down to a low level. It will remain low until around the time of ovulation. This low level usually ranges from 96 to 97.4 degrees, although for some women it can be somewhat higher. After ovulation it will rise to a higher level, usually from 3/10 (three-tenths or .3) of a degree to 1.0 degree higher than the previous low temperature.

This rise in temperature, after it has remained high for at least 3 days, is proof that an egg has been released from the ovary.

Basal body temperature will remain high for about 12 to 16 days. Menstrual bleeding usually occurs when the temperature begins to fall. If your basal body temperature

remains high longer than 20 days and sexual intercourse occurred during a fertile time, this can be a reliable sign of pregnancy.

Is it correct to say that ovulation takes place the day before the temperature rise? NO! It usually does, but it can take place the day of the rise, the day after the rise, or several days before the temperature rise. That is how it tells us that the egg **has been** released.

Cervix

The third primary fertility sign is changes in the cervix. Although cervical changes do not have to be observed to determine days of fertility and infertility, they can provide valuable information about your fertility pattern.

During the menstrual flow your cervix is low in the vaginal canal. The area surrounding its opening will be soft and will have widened to allow for the menstrual flow.

When your period ends, your cervix will usually be located low in the vaginal canal. If you touch it with your finger, you can feel that your cervix is closer to your vaginal opening. The way it feels also changes. It becomes firm, feeling like the tip of a nose or a small rubber ball, and the opening is closed.

For a woman who has not had a vaginal delivery, the opening is like a dimple; whereas the woman who has delivered vaginally may notice a cervical opening that feels irregular and wide. Also, if you have delivered children vaginally, you may have relaxed support of the uterus, making it difficult to feel the rising and lowering of the cervix.

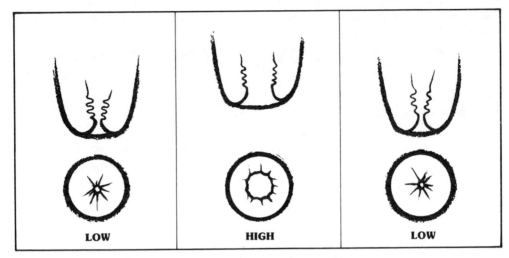

| LOW | HIGH | LOW |

Figure 15 —Changes of the Cervix

As ovulation approaches, the rising estrogen levels cause the cervix to move away from the vaginal opening, making it more difficult to touch in the vaginal canal. Also, the cervical opening begins to widen and the area surrounding it softens. The texture of the cervix now can be compared to the softness of the lips. This rising and opening of the cervix occur to help sperm travel into the uterus.

After ovulation, the rising progesterone levels cause the cervix once again to lower in the vaginal canal and become firmer, and the cervical opening becomes smaller. These changes help prevent sperm from entering the uterus.

Is it correct to say that ovulation took place when the cervix was at its highest, most soft and open time? NO! The cervix warns you that the egg is preparing to leave the ovary. Cervical changes cannot tell you the exact day ovulation takes place.

Just as some women have noticed their normally changing mucus signs without connecting them to their fertility patterns, some are familiar with their cervical changes. For example, inserting a tampon or having intercourse in certain positions can be uncomfortable when the cervix is in its low position.

TO REVIEW:

The main fertility signs

> *cervical mucus*
> *basal body temperature*
> *the cervix*

enable you to make accurate and sensible choices concerning your fertility. Since they help you determine your fertile and infertile days, you will have information that can lead to an excellent way of planning sexual intercourse to either prevent or achieve pregnancy.

CHAPTER VI

THE MINOR ONES
Secondary Fertility Signs

Nature has given you signs that will enable you to know when the egg is about to be released as well as when it has been released and when it can no longer be fertilized. Though you won't be able to know the exact time and day of ovulation, by observing your fertility signs you can accurately determine the days when you can or cannot become pregnant.

Remember, you have 3 primary fertility signs:

1. **Cervical mucus serves as a sign of approaching ovulation and can give you an idea of when ovulation has taken place.**
2. **Basal body temperature can tell you when ovulation has taken place.**
3. **Cervical changes can provide you with additional information about the approach and end of ovulation.**

Remember these facts:

- *The first day of the menstrual cycle begins with the first day of bleeding.*
- *The cycle ends the day before the next bleeding begins.*
- *The menstrual cycle is your fertility cycle.*
- *Ovulation occurs about 12 to 16 days before menstrual bleeding.*
- *Ovulation can take place at any time after a menstrual cycle begins.*
- *An egg is able to be fertilized for 12 to 24 hours after ovulation.*
- *Sperm are capable of fertilizing the egg up to 5 days when fertile cervical mucus is present.*
- *The primary fertility signs coincide with all this information.*

These facts make up the major principles for the use of fertility signs to prevent or achieve a pregnancy.

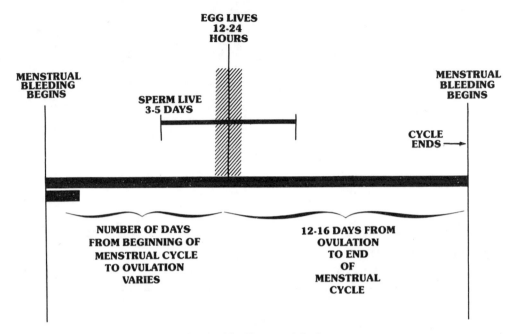

EGG LIVES
12-24
HOURS

MENSTRUAL
BLEEDING
BEGINS

MENSTRUAL
BLEEDING
BEGINS

SPERM LIVE
3-5 DAYS

CYCLE
ENDS →

NUMBER OF DAYS
FROM BEGINNING OF
MENSTRUAL CYCLE
TO OVULATION
VARIES

12-16 DAYS FROM
OVULATION
TO END
OF
MENSTRUAL
CYCLE

Figure 16—Menstrual Cycle

Other changes may occur in a woman's body around the time of ovulation that provide additional information about her own unique fertility pattern. These are called secondary fertility signs.

They are useful signs. But since not all women experience them, they are not as dependable for determining the time of ovulation as cervical mucus, basal body temperature and the cervix.

About 12 to 16 days after the release of the egg, if pregnancy does not occur, estrogen and progesterone levels decrease, causing the menstrual flow to begin. The decrease in these hormones at the end of the menstrual cycle may cause many bodily changes known as premenstrual symptoms.

As menstruation nears, the body's oil-producing glands secrete more oil, causing an increase in acne and oily skin. Cramping, leg aches and backaches can occur. Your body may hold more fluid, causing breast tenderness. You may also experience itching of the nipples, headaches and mood changes. Some women notice an increase or decrease in sexual feelings at this time.

These premenstrual symptoms*, known as the premenstrual syndrome, can cause some women to feel very uncomfortable for a day or more before their menstrual bleeding begins and can seriously affect their lives in a negative way.

*See the Bibliography for books that discuss premenstrual symptoms in detail as well as various ways to treat them.

There are different theories about the causes of premenstrual syndrome as well as the treatments. Some people feel that the use of progesterone is the answer. Others believe that treatment should include the use of specific vitamins combined with special diets, exercises, and various stress-reducing techniques. If you find that you, or someone you know, is experiencing certain physical and/or emotional changes 1 to 14 days before menstruation, you should know that help is available. You can read information about premenstrual syndrome and discuss it with your physician as well as contact organizations that have been formed to help women with this problem.

Just as these signs tell you menstruation is going to begin, other bodily changes may occur that can help you know when your ovulation time is near.

As ovulation approaches, the body's oil-producing glands secrete less oil. This causes a decrease in oily skin and for some women a clearer complexion. Some women also find their bodies begin to "hold water," called fluid retention. Fluid retention causes a slight bloated feeling, slight breast tenderness and even irritability. These feelings are not as severe as those experienced premenstrually and usually last for only a day or two.

Some women notice an increase in energy during the days leading up to ovulation. In fact, some women even experience a sharper sense of vision, smell and taste as their ovulation approaches.

A dull ache or pain may occur in the pelvic area shortly before, during or shortly after ovulation. This pain or ache may last a few moments or a few days. It may occur on one side of the pelvic area or on both

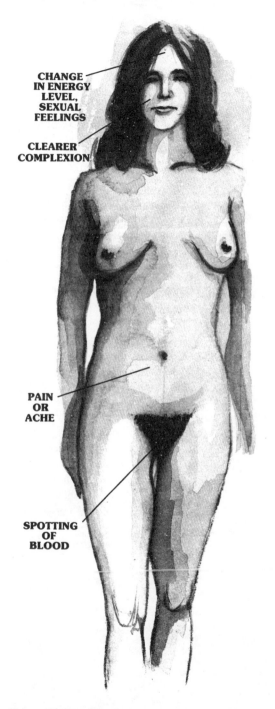

CHANGE IN ENERGY LEVEL, SEXUAL FEELINGS

CLEARER COMPLEXION

PAIN OR ACHE

SPOTTING OF BLOOD

Figure 17—Possible Secondary Fertility Signs as ovulation nears

sides. It may travel down one or both legs and even around to the lower back. This pain may be accompanied by spotting or a light flow of blood.

Around the time of ovulation, some women notice an increase in sexual feelings. Others experience no change or even a decrease in sexual feelings.

Some women experience all of these changes while others experience only a few. For those women who experience them, these changes can be very helpful when learning about their own special fertility patterns.

A word about primary and secondary fertility signs.

It would be wonderful if there were a way for you to determine the exact day the egg is released from the ovary. Unfortunately, it must be remembered that at the present time there is none. Yet if fertility signs are observed carefully, you can learn the approximate time of ovulation. Through the observations of fertility signs, you can tell when the time of ovulation is approaching as well as when it has occurred. Therefore, you will see and feel the beginning of your fertile time early enough in the menstrual cycle to prevent or achieve a pregnancy.

TO REVIEW:

During the fertility cycle you will experience two types of signs or signals — three primary signs and several secondary signs.

Primary Changes

  Cervical mucus
  Basal body temperature
  Cervix

Possible Secondary Changes

  Condition of skin and hair
  Water retention
  Aches, pain
  Sensitivity in skin and breasts
  Energy levels and mood
  Sexual feelings

It is important for you to keep a record of as many bodily changes as possible. By keeping a chart of your individual pattern of fertility signs, you will be able to gain a clearer understanding of the fertile and infertile times of your menstrual cycle. It will also increase your awareness of your own normal bodily changes.

CHAPTER VII

OBSERVING THE WAY TO AWARENESS

The first step in learning about your own fertility pattern is to observe it carefully. To accomplish this, we recommend that you use as many fertility signs as you are comfortable with to prevent pregnancy. Since you will be establishing a new habit, learning accurate information and developing your fertility awareness, it is important that you check your fertility signs every day until you feel you have learned your fertility pattern.

You need only 10 to 15 minutes each day to observe fertility signs accurately. As you gain experience, you will get better and better, decreasing the time spent. In fact, once you learn your own fertility cycle and enter the non-fertile part of your menstrual cycle, it is not necessary to check your signs for the remainder of that cycle.

Checking your fertility signs can be compared to the daily habit of brushing your teeth. It's done automatically and regularly and takes a few minutes. You pick up the toothbrush, squeeze the tube of toothpaste and brush your teeth — without thinking. Placing a thermometer under your tongue and looking at cervical mucus and other signs can also become part of your daily routine. Before long it's habit and you do it without giving it a second thought.

Cervical Mucus Observation

When you wake up in the morning, before you bathe and wash them away, you should find out about your cervical mucus and vaginal sensations. Ask yourself this question; "Does the vagina feel wet or dry?" What you feel on the outside of your vagina depends on whether mucus is present and on the quality of this mucus. For example, wet mucus will make the outside of the vagina feel wet. And non-wet mucus will make the outside of the vagina feel dry. An absence of mucus also causes the outside of the vagina to feel dry. Once you have decided how the outside of the vagina feels, the next step is external checking.

External Checking. External checking is a technique that enables you to *see* if mucus is present, as well as assess the quality, color and amount of mucus.

THERE ARE THREE STEPS TO EXTERNAL CHECKING:

1. Take a piece of folded white toilet tissue and wipe the outside of the vaginal opening.
2. Next, look at the toilet tissue and answer these questions:

   - Is there any mucus on the toilet tissue?
   - If so, what color is it?
   - How much mucus is on the toilet tissue?

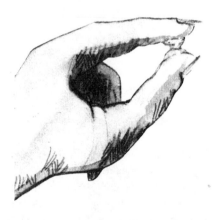

Figure 18—Slowly Part Fingers

3. Then check how the mucus feels.

   - Take a sample of the mucus between two fingers to determine how it feels.

- Draw the fingers *slowly* apart to see if the mucus stretches or just forms little peaks.
- Does the mucus feel dry, pasty and crumbly or does it feel wet? Does it feel stretchy and slippery?
- *Your cervical mucus should be checked several times throughout the day — at least once in the morning, afternoon and evening. However, the more often you check your mucus, the better. Many women find it convenient to check their cervical mucus each time they go to the bathroom.*

TO REVIEW:

Vaginal Sensations

- *How does the outside of the vaginal area feel?*
  - *Is it wet feeling?*
  - *Is it dry feeling?*

Cervical Mucus

- *Collect some mucus.*
- *Look at the mucus.*
  - *Is it clear or cloudy?*
  - *Is it creamy or lumpy?*
- *Feel the mucus.*
  - *Is it slippery?*
  - *Is it pasty?*
  - *Is it crumbly?*
- *Try to stretch the mucus between your fingers.*

Vaginal feelings are also called vaginal sensations. They are not experienced by touching the vaginal area with the fingers. They are feelings a woman mentally "tunes into." While walking, sitting, and lying down, a woman needs to ask herself, "Do I feel wet or dry?" Through continuous practice, assessing vaginal sensations becomes easier and easier. In fact, some women become so experienced with evaluating their vaginal sensations they know which type of mucus they are producing without even using the external mucus checking technique. Even if this level of experience is gained, we still strongly suggest that the woman continue with regular mucus checking. Combining knowledge of vaginal sensations and cervical mucus is the ideal way to go when using this knowledge to prevent pregnancy.

HELPFUL HINTS FOR EXTERNAL CHECKING

Kegel Exercise

No doubt you have had to go to the bathroom when there was no bathroom in sight. To prevent an "accident," you tightly squeezed those muscles that enable you to prevent the flow of urine. These muscles surrounding the vagina are called the pubbococcygeal (PC) muscles. The Kegel Exercise is the tightening and relaxing of these PC muscles. To perform it you should squeeze the muscles tightly for a few seconds, then relax them. Repeat the tightening and relaxing of the muscles 10 times in a row. This helps push any mucus at the cervix down to the vaginal opening. The Kegel Exercise is excellent for keeping your vaginal muscles in shape. Not only does the exercise aid in pushing mucus down the vaginal canal, but many women feel that it also helps to increase sexual pleasure for themselves and their partners.

Other excellent times to check cervical mucus are following physical exercise or bowel movements. As with the Kegel Exercise, these activities cause the mucus to travel down to the vaginal opening.

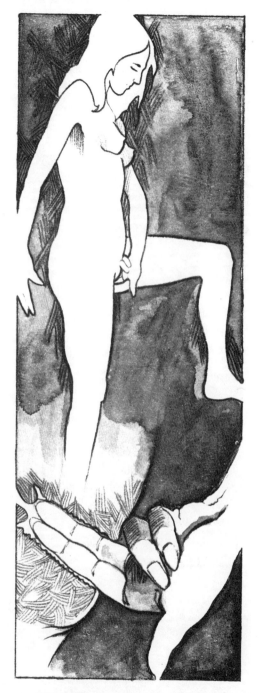

Figure 19—Checking of the Cervix

INTERNAL CHECKING

Some women choose to observe their mucus changes by taking a sample of the mucus directly from the cervical opening (see page 76). There is no evidence to suggest that internal checking is more accurate than external checking. However, if a woman wishes to observe her mucus in this manner, she will need to learn the difference between normal vaginal secretions and her cervical mucus.

Observation of the Cervix

Checking cervical changes can be done at the same time that you check your cervical mucus.

The changes in the cervix are observed by taking the following steps:

1. Wash the hands before checking the cervix to avoid the possibility of vaginal infection.
2. Insert one or two fingers into the vaginal opening.
3. Apply gentle pressure to allow the finger to pass up the vaginal canal. When the finger has reached the back of the vagina, the cervix can be felt. It is smooth, round and feels firmer than the tissue of the vagina that surrounds it.

4. As the cervix is being felt, answer the following questions:
   - Is it easy or difficult to reach the cervix? In other words, is the cervix low or high in the vaginal canal?
   - Does the cervix feel firm like the tip of a nose? Does it feel soft like the lips of a mouth?
   - Does the opening feel closed like a small dimple? Does it feel open like a small hole?

5. The cervix should be felt throughout the day, if possible. If this is not possible, it should be checked at least once in the morning and once in the evening.

6. Squatting or placing one foot on a stool are good positions for cervical checking. The same position should be used each time the cervix is checked.

Although the combination of cervical mucus and basal body temperature changes provides enough information to identify the fertile and infertile phases accurately, some women have found observing cervical changes to be valuable for helping them determine these phases.

TO REVIEW:

Cervical Changes

- *Relax and find the best position.*
- *Feel the opening of the cervix.*
- *Is the cervix difficult or easy to reach (high or low)?*
- *Is it soft or firm?*
- *Is it opening or closing as compared to the last check?*

notes:

Basal Body Temperature Observation

The third primary fertility sign to observe is your basal body temperature (BBT). You should use a basal body temperature thermometer. This is a special thermometer that is marked in one-tenths of degrees, allowing greater accuracy in measuring basal body temperature changes. The fever thermometer is different because it is marked in two-tenths of degrees. Since the BBT thermometer gives a more accurate reading of the basal body temperature, you will achieve better results by using one. If you are unable to purchase a BBT thermometer, a fever thermometer may do.

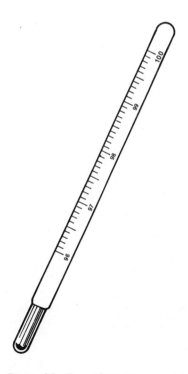

Figure 20—Basal Body Thermometer

This is how you take your temperature:

1. Take your temperature as soon as you awaken, before you get out of bed or engage in any kind of activity.
2. Take your temperature either orally (under your tongue), rectally (in your rectum), or vaginally (in your vagina) for 5 minutes. Since it is important to be consistent, use the same method each time you take your temperature.

Many women find that taking their temperature orally is most convenient. However, sinus or breathing problems may require that you take your temperature vaginally or rectally.

It must be remembered that temperatures taken vaginally and rectally are about 1.0 full degree higher than oral temperatures. Therefore, taking your temperature rectally or vaginally one day and orally another day will not provide an accurate account of the temperature pattern.

If for some reason you have to take your temperature differently one day, be sure to make a note of this on your fertility awareness chart.

3. Once the 5 minutes is up, read the thermometer and record your temperature on the chart. If you feel like going back to sleep after taking your temperature, put the thermometer in a safe place and read it later. Be careful not to place it near a heater, a lamp or on a sunny ledge since the reading could easily be affected by the heat.
4. Once the temperature is recorded, the thermometer should be shaken down and placed safely in its case, available for use the next day.

5. Take your temperature about the same time every day. This guarantees a more accurate temperature pattern throughout the menstrual cycle. However, if you oversleep one day or need to awaken earlier than usual another day, take your temperature when you wake up and record it. An occasional early or late temperature can be adjusted.

6. When the temperature is recorded daily, it is important to make note of any activity that may cause the temperature to be unusual. For example, taking the temperature in a different manner than usual, drinking alcohol, taking a medication or a drug, awakening later or earlier than usual or a restless night's sleep may make the temperature abnormally high or low.

   These events may not cause a change, but as long as they have been recorded, if they do affect your temperature, you can make adjustments for them.

7. If the mercury in the thermometer is between 2 lines, the lower of the 2 temperatures is recorded. For example, if the mercury reads between 97.1 and 97.2 degrees, the 97.1 reading is recorded as the temperature for the day.

8. Regardless of how the temperature is taken, you should try not to fall asleep with the thermometer in place. Rolling over may break it. The thermometer could also fall out of place, causing an inaccurate reading for the day.

Instructions for Using the BBT Thermometer

1. Place the rounded mercury end of the thermometer under your tongue. Keep your lips closed over the thermometer.

or

2. Place the first half inch of the thermometer in the rectum. (Putting vaseline or an oil on the tip of the thermometer makes inserting a rectal thermometer more comfortable.)

or

3. Place the first half inch of the thermometer into the vaginal opening. (Do not use any type of lubrication — oil or jelly — since these can affect the mucus check.)

TO REVIEW:

Basal Body Temperature

- *Use a BBT Thermometer.*
- *Take your temperature just after you wake up.*
- *Do not engage in any activity before you take your temperature — no smoking, eating, drinking or sexual activity.*
- *Take your temperature at the same time each day.*
- *Keep the thermometer in place for 5 minutes.*

These temperature-taking instructions should be followed as closely as possible. Yet, unexpected situations can occur — the need to go to the bathroom, tend a child or answer a phone call. In these situations, you should still take your temperature as soon as you are able to.

Remember, your basal body temperature is the body temperature at rest, unaffected by activity — drinking, smoking, eating, etc. For the woman who works evenings or nights, the temperature should be taken after her usual time of sleeping.

For some women, the basal body temperature is the fertility sign most difficult to observe because it requires awakening at about the same time every day. On the other hand, some women have found that taking their temperature is not difficult.

notes:

It is a good time to relax and plan their day's activities. It has helped others to establish a routine of getting up earlier so that they have time for breakfast or an exercise routine they have wanted to enjoy.

ONE MORE WORD ABOUT THE OBSERVATION OF FERTILITY SIGNS

If you feel that observing your fertility signs might be difficult for you, remember that once you feel comfortable and familiar with your fertility pattern, *you will not have to take your temperature and check your cervical mucus and cervix every day.* In fact, as soon as you enter your definitely infertile time, you can put the thermometer away and stop checking your temperature as well as the other fertility signs until your next menstrual cycle begins.

notes:

CHAPTER VIII

CHARTING THE WAY TO AWARENESS

- The first step in learning about your fertility pattern is to observe your fertility signs.
- The next step is to record them on the fertility awareness chart. You will then have a visual story of each fertiltiy cycle. (See Figure 21.)

Recording Cervical Mucus on the Fertility Awareness Chart

The following symbols are used for recording cervical mucus changes:

1. **✳** represents menstrual bleeding.
2. **D** represents dry days. These are the days when mucus is not present and the outside of the vagina feels dry.
3. **M** represents non-wet mucus. These are the days when sticky, pasty — but not wet — mucus is present and the outside of the vagina feels dry.
4. **Ⓜ** represents wet mucus. These are the days when any form of wet-feeling mucus is present and the outside of the vagina feels wet. Sometimes a wet sensation will be noticed on the outside of the vagina, but the mucus is not yet visible on the outside. In this situation the day is still considered an **Ⓜ**, a wet mucus day.

5. **⊗** represents the one day that is the *last day* of wet-feeling mucus and a wet vaginal sensation. This final day is called the *peak day*. It is important to be on the lookout for this last day, especially if you are using your fertility signs as a way of preventing a pregnancy. (The peak day rule will be explained in Chapter 9).

In addition to using these symbols, it can also be helpful to write down mucus descriptions in the "notes" column on the chart. These descriptions would include the color, amount and quality of the mucus.

Recording Cervical Changes on the Fertility Awareness Chart

Cervical changes are recorded in the following ways:

1. A small closed circle placed in the lower left-hand corner of the box represents a low closed cervix. |•|
2. A larger circle represents the cervix as its opening enlarges. Every day the opening feels larger, the circle becomes more open. |o|

3. As the cervix becomes higher in the vaginal canal, the circles are placed higher in the boxes. O
4. **S** represents a soft cervix. Os
5. **F** represents a firm cervix. F
   S and **F** are also recorded in the boxes.

SPECIAL NOTE:

When the fertility signs are not the same throughout the day, *the most fertile sign of the day is to be recorded.* For example, if you have no mucus in the morning but notice a small amount of pasty mucus in the evening, the small amount of pasty mucus is recorded as the mucus of the day.

If you feel wet, creamy mucus in the morning and pasty, sticky, non-wet mucus in the evening, the wet, creamy mucus is recorded as the mucus of the day. If you feel the cervix in a low position in the morning and afternoon, but by evening it feels higher, the higher cervix observation is recorded.

Recording Basal Body Temperature (BBT) on the Fertility Awareness Chart

BBT changes are recorded in the following way:

1. Basal body temperature (BBT) must be recorded accurately in the temperature columns on the fertility awareness chart.
2. Circle the temperature on the chart that is the same as your temperature for the day.
3. Connect each circle with a straight line. This makes the changes of the temperature clear to see.

4. The time you have chosen to take your temperature each day is written in the "usual time" space on the left-hand side of the chart.
5. If you awaken earlier or later than usual or experience anything else that you think might affect an accurate temperature reading, record this in the "notes" column.

Recording Secondary Fertility Signs on the Fertility Awareness Chart

Secondary fertility signs are recorded in the following way:

1. All physical and/or emotional changes experienced during each menstrual cycle should be recorded in the "notes" column.
2. These changes are recorded on the exact day that they are experienced.

Everything and anything you feel should be written down to help you learn about your own special fertility cycle. The more information you record, the less you will need to remember, and the greater will be the rewards and discoveries you experience as your body undergoes its changes during the fertility cycle.

The key to every facet of the information in this book is that it is your body talking to you. Your body is letting you know what is occurring with your fertility cycle — a pattern of events and changes that will provide for you a personal profile, a profile that speaks a silent but powerful personal language: The language of fertility.

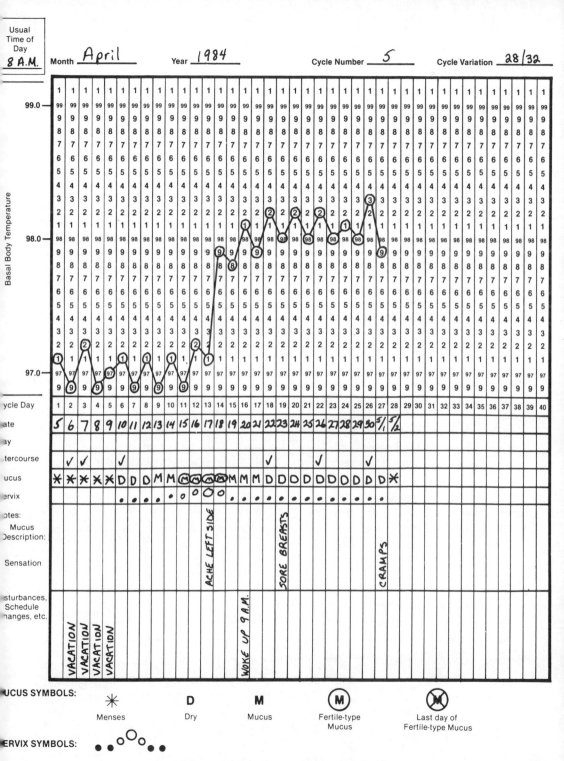

FIGURE 21—RECORDING FERTILITY SIGNS

Figure 21 is an example of how to complete the fertility awareness chart.

The usual time of day the temperature is taken and the month and year of the cycle being recorded should be noted. In this case the usual time of temperature taking is 8:00 a.m. and the month and year of the cycle is April, 1982. The cycle number should be filled in with the number of the present cycle being observed which is cycle number 5. Cycle variation represents the number of days in the shortest and longest cycle. In this chart, the number of days in the shortest menstrual cycle was 28 and the number of days in the longest menstrual cycle was 32. The cycle variation notation should always reflect the lengths of the 6 most recent menstrual cycles. If a woman does not know the lengths of her 6 most recent menstrual cycles or if she has just discontinued taking birth control pills, just had a baby, or experienced any situation that stopped ovulation, she should record her cycle lengths as she experiences them. The fertility signs the woman chooses to observe are recorded on a daily basis as well as any other descriptions of mucus, vaginal sensations and secondary fertility signs. Of course, any changes in lifestyle should be noted in the appropriate columns at the bottom of the chart. As you can see, on cycle days 3 through 6, a vacation was noted. Though a vacation may not change the menstrual cycle, it may, so it is noted just in case.

To review this chart:

The woman had knowledge of her previous 4 menstrual cycles. This was the fifth cycle she was charting. The shortest cycle of her previous 4 cycles was 28 days long. The longest cycle was 32 days long. Therefore, her cycle variation up to this point is 28/32. The next chart she records will have cycle number 6 noted. Since this cycle was 27 days long, her cycle variation on her next chart would be noted 27/32 instead of the previous 28/32. She usually takes her temperature at 8:00 a.m. This is marked in the "usual time" space. In the notes column, she recorded aching on her left side on the 13th day of her menstrual cycle. On the 27th day of her menstrual cycle, she experienced menstrual cramps which she also noted. This woman recorded the fact that she awoke later than usual on cycle day 12. She also recorded the days she had intercourse by placing a "✔" in the column marked intercourse. Please note that the more complete a chart is, the better able a woman is to apply the natural family planning rules accurately.

CHAPTER IX

PUTTING IT ALL TOGETHER THE NATURAL FAMILY PLANNING WAY
Rules for Avoiding Pregnancy

The natural family planning rules for avoiding pregnancy are directions that show you how to determine the days you can have intercourse with a minimal chance of pregnancy.

When these rules are accurately applied to fertility signs and followed correctly, they can provide you with an extremely safe and effective way to avoid an unplanned pregnancy.

We have 2 sets of natural family planning rules:

1. *One set is used to determine the infertile days before ovulation.*
2. *The second set is used to determine the infertile days after ovulation.*

Together the 2 sets of rules enable you to divide your menstrual cycle into 3 parts or 3 phases:

1. *Phase I, the calculated infertile time.*
2. *Phase II, the fertile time.*
3. *Phase III, the absolutely infertile time.*

During the CALCULATED INFERTILE PHASE I (CIP), intercourse may occur with a very small chance of pregnancy.

During the FERTILE PHASE II, if intercourse does take place, the chance of pregnancy is great.

In the ABSOLUTELY INFERTILE PHASE III (AIP), intercourse can occur with almost no chance of pregnancy.

Natural Family Planning Rules Used to Determine the Absolutely Infertile Phase III

There are 3 rules which you can use to determine when the absolutely infertile phase begins. These are:

Thermal Shift Rule
Peak Day Rule
Cervix Closing Rule

Thermal Shift Rule

The thermal shift rule is the rule that is applied to the basal body temperature. It is called the thermal shift rule because you will be on the lookout for a shift in temperature. A shift is a change (a rise) from the low temperatures occurring before ovulation to the higher temperatures occurring after ovulation. In other words, the basal body temperature will shift upward at some point after the egg has been released. (If you recall, the heat-producing hormone progesterone, which is released after ovulation, causes the temperature to rise.)

You will notice that at some time during your menstrual cycle, your temperature will rise from 2/10 (two-tenths or .2) of a degree to 1.0 full degree higher than the previous low temperatures. A simple statement of the thermal shift rule is that once 3 high temperatures are recorded, the absolutely infertile phase begins. Actually there is a bit more to the rule than that. *The 3 high temperatures must also be above the coverline.*

Coverline. A coverline is a line drawn across the basal body temperature chart which will help you determine accurately the beginning of the absolutely infertile time. *To draw a coverline you need to look at the 6 temperatures recorded immediately before the temperature shifts to a higher level.* This means that starting with the day *before* the temperature shift, you count back 6 temperatures in a row. Then draw a coverline which is 1/10 of a degree above the highest of the 6 temperatures. For example, if the highest of your 6 temperatures before the rise is 97.4, you would add 1/10 of a degree to 97.4. This gives you a coverline of 97.5.

Remember that the egg will only live for 24 hours unless it is fertilized. Waiting to resume intercourse until the evening of the third day allows sufficient time for the release and life span of one, perhaps two, eggs. If an egg is no longer present, there can be no pregnancy!

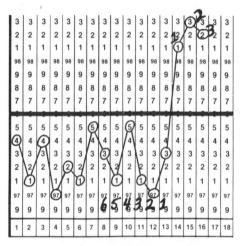

Figure 22—The Thermal Shift Rule

In Figure 22 — the temperature shifted to 98.1 on cycle day 14. To draw the coverline, we first look at the 6 temperatures in a row recorded right before the day of the shift. Next, we find the highest of the 6 temperatures. In this case it is 97.5. Finally, by adding 1/10 of a degree to 97.5, we can draw the coverline at 97.6. Waiting for 3 temperatures in a row to be recorded above the coverline gives us an absolutely infertile phase beginning on the evening of cycle day 16.

Caution:

If any 1 of the 3 temperatures falls on or below the coverline, it can be a sign that ovulation has not yet taken place. Therefore, wait until the temperatures rise back above the coverline and then apply the 3-day count again.

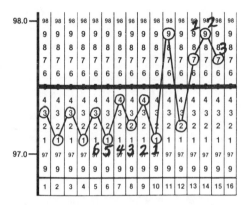

Figure 23—Identifying the True Thermal Shift

In Figure 23 — the temperature shifted to 97.9 on cycle day 11. The coverline was drawn at 97.5, which is 1/10 of a degree above the highest of the 6 previous low temperatures. As you can see, the temperature dropped back down below the coverline. Therefore, we have to wait until the true shift in temperature takes place to determine the beginning of the absolutely infertile phase. The temperature rises again on cycle day 13. We know it is the true thermal shift because the temperature stays above the line for 3 days in a row. Therefore, in this example the absolutely infertile phase begins on the evening of cycle day 15.

False High Rises. Occasionally, around the time of ovulation, you may observe a rise in temperature and assume it is your thermal shift. However, instead of remaining above the coverline for 3 consecutive days, the temperature may fall back on or below it. Therefore, the temperature rise was for a reason other than ovulation. This is called a false high rise. A false high rise can be caused

by oversleeping one day or by experiencing one of the situations discussed in Chapter 7 that can cause an unusual temperature rise. False high rises, as we have stated, cannot be used when applying the thermal shift rule. Always use only those high temperatures which reflect accurate normal basal body temperatures.

A false high temperature can also occur early in the menstrual cycle. However, this will not prevent you from correctly applying the thermal shift rule. For example, if one of the 6 temperatures before the rise is high instead of low, it would not be used to determine the

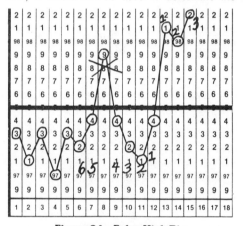

Figure 24—False High Rise

In Figure 24 — the temperature rises on cycle day 8. Because the rise had taken place in the early part of Jane's menstrual cycle, before she usually experiences her thermal shift, she knew this rise was probably not her real thermal shift. She also overslept that morning and took her temperature a couple of hours later than usual. (Though she could be experiencing an unexpected early ovulation, she was not producing any cervical mucus. If she were ovulating early, she would be able to observe the early warning sign of mucus.) She continued to take her temperature and found that it shifted on cycle day 13. She drew her coverline 1/10 of a degree above the highest of the 6 temperatures recorded before the thermal shift. Since the temperature on cycle day 8 was unusually high, it would not be used as one of the 6 temperatures. Jane "skipped over" this temperature and continued to count back until she had the 6 temperatures needed to draw the coverline.

—47—

coverline. Just skip this unusually high temperature and continue to count back until you have 6 low temperatures to use.

The only situation to be concerned about is when there are more than 2 high temperatures during the 6 days before the shift. This can reflect improper temperature taking or perhaps an unusual menstrual cycle. If this should happen, we suggest continuing abstinence until you can discuss this irregular basal body temperature with someone very experienced in the use of fertility signs.

TO REVIEW:

1. *Be on the lookout for a shift in temperature from 2/10 of a degree to 1.0 full degree higher than the previous 6 temperatures. The 6 temperatures used are the ones which occur immediately before the rise.*
2. *Draw the coverline 1/10 of a degree above the highest of the 6 temperatures.*
3. *Wait for 3 days in a row of high temperatures above the coverline.*
4. *The evening of the third day of high temperatures is the beginning of the absolutely infertile phase and intercourse can be resumed until the next menstrual flow begins.*
5. *You can put your thermometer away after the beginning of the absolutely infertile phase.*

Slow-Rising Temperatures. Some women may find that their temperatures shift slowly over a period of a few days instead of shifting 2/10 of a degree or more in one day. These slow-rising temperatures can make it difficult to determine the exact day the shift takes place. In this situation the coverline is

determined differently so that the thermal shift rule can be accurately applied.

The coverline is drawn 1/10 of a degree above the highest of the *first 10 temperatures* of the menstrual cycle. (Temperatures which are high during the menstrual flow should not be used when determining the coverline.) For example, if the highest of the first 10 temperatures is 97.6, the coverline would be drawn at 97.7 degrees.

SLOW SHIFTING
THERMAL SHIFT RULE

The Absolutely Infertile Phase (AIP) begins on the evening of the fifth consecutive day of temperatures recorded above the coverline.

Since the temperature is rising slowly, the 5-day temperature count ensures that an egg is no longer present to be fertilized.

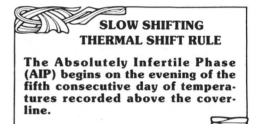

Figure 25—The Thermal Shift Rule for the Slow Shifting Temperature Pattern

In Figure 25 — you can see that the temperatures are rising slowly, making it difficult to determine the exact day of the temperature shift. Drawing a coverline above the highest of the first 10 temperatures is a simple way to handle this situation. The coverline is drawn here at 97.7, which is 1/10 of a degree above 97.6, the highest temperature during the first 10 days. Since the fifth temperature in a row recorded above the coverline begins the absolutely infertile phase, in this example it begins on the evening of cycle day 16.

Caution:

If any one of the 5 temperatures falls on or below the coverline, it can be a sign that ovulation has not yet taken place. Therefore, wait until the temperatures rise back above the coverline and then apply the 5-day count.

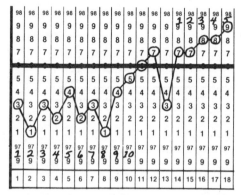

Figure 26—Identifying the True Thermal Shift Slow-Rising

In Figure 26 — the temperature appears to begin to rise slowly on cycle day 11. Because of this slow rise, Susan draws her coverline at 97.5, which is 1/10 of a degree above the highest of the first 10 temperatures. On cycle day 13 the temperature falls below the coverline. Because of this, she must wait for the temperature to rise back above the coverline to apply the thermal shift rule. Since we are using the thermal shift rule for the slow-rising temperature pattern, the absolutely infertile phase begins on the evening of the fifth day of temperatures recorded above the coverline. In this example, it begins on the evening of cycle day 18.

TO REVIEW:

1. *Draw the coverline 1/10 of a degree above the highest of the first 10 temperatures of the menstrual cycle.*
2. *The evening of the fifth day of temperatures recorded above the coverline is the beginning of the absolutely infertile phase.*

Peak Day Rule

The peak day rule is the rule applied to the cervical mucus. It is called the peak day rule because the peak day must be identified in order to apply this rule.

As you recall, at some point after the menstrual flow ends, cervical mucus will be observed. As ovulation nears, this mucus will become very wet, slippery and stretchy, causing a wet sensation at the outside of the vaginal area. At some point after ovulation, the mucus will lose most if not all of its wet quality, and the wet vaginal sensation will no longer be present. *The last day of the wet vaginal sensation and very wet mucus is the peak day.* To identify the peak day you will be looking for the first day the wet vaginal sensation is no longer present and the mucus feels significantly drier. (Some women notice that they stop having mucus for the remainder of the menstrual cycle.) As you can see, the peak day can be identified only after it has taken place. For example, you may experience wet mucus and a wet vaginal sensation Monday through Friday; then on Saturday you observe a mucus that is no longer wet or considerably less wet than it has been, and the wet vaginal sensation is gone. This means that Friday, the last day of your wet sensation and a significantly drier feeling mucus, is your peak day.

PEAK DAY RULE
The Absolutely Infertile Phase (AIP) begins on the evening of the fourth consecutive day of non-wet mucus and/or dry days after the peak day.

As you probably have noticed, we continuously reinforce vaginal sensations. Remember that the vaginal sensations experienced are dependent upon the quality of the mucus present. Wet mucus causes a wet vaginal sensation, and a total absence of mucus or sticky, non-wet mucus causes a dry vaginal sensation.

If you feel a wet sensation but don't see wet mucus, your peak day has not yet occurred. You have experienced the last day of wetness — the peak day — only when both the mucus and vaginal sensation demonstrate dryness.

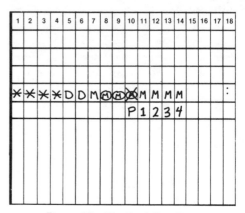

Figure 28—The Peak Day Rule

In Figure 28 — on cycle day 11 Marlene no longer experienced wet vaginal sensations and her mucus felt considerably drier than it had on cycle days 8, 9, and 10. Because of this she could mark cycle day 10, the last wet day, as her peak day. Marlene could then apply the peak day rule because she experienced 4 non-wet days in a row after her peak day. Her absolutely infertile phase began on the evening of cycle day 14.

Remember:

Ovulation can occur any time from a few days before the peak day to a few days after the peak day. Waiting until the evening of the fourth day to resume intercourse provides sufficient time for the release and life span of the egg. When the absolutely infertile phase begins, you no longer need to observe your mucus.

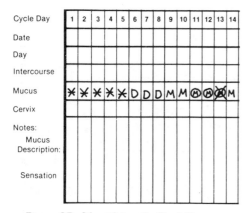

Figure 27—Identifying the Peak Day

In Figure 27 — Joanne has recorded 5 days of menstrual bleeding. Once the bleeding ended, she began observing for mucus. On cycle days 6, 7, and 8, because no mucus was observed and a dry vaginal sensation was felt, these days were recorded as dry days. On cycle days 9 and 10 she experienced a non-wet quality mucus with a dry vaginal sensation. Joanne began producing wet-quality mucus on cycle day 11. These wet days continued until cycle day 13. On cycle day 14 she noticed that her wet sensations were no longer present. She felt a dry sensation and non-wet mucus. At this point she was able to go back to the last day of wet-quality mucus and wet sensations and mark it as her peak day. Placing an X through the circled M represented the peak day for that cycle.

Once the peak day is determined, the rule can be applied.

Caution:

Occasionally a woman experiences the reappearance of wet mucus after she has identified what she believed to be her peak day. She will know it was not her peak day because instead of having 4 non-wet days in a row, wet mucus reappears. If this happens, abstinence should be continued until the true peak day is identified and the wetness is absent for 4 days in a row.

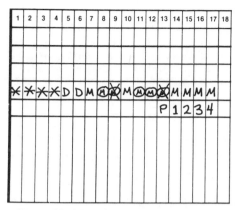

Figure 29—Identifying the True Peak Day

In Figure 29 — Ruth thought her peak day occurred on cycle day 9 since on cycle day 10 she experienced a drier-feeling mucus with dry vaginal sensations. However, while waiting for the 4 non-wet days to pass, she noticed a reappearance of wet mucus. She realized that either she made an error in identifying her peak day or perhaps was ovulating later than usual. She continued to abstain and waited until her wet mucus production stopped. She then identified a peak day on cycle day 13. This time she was correct because she then experienced non-wet mucus days with dry vaginal sensations for 4 days in a row. Therefore, according to the peak day rule, her absolutely infertile phase began the evening of cycle day 17.

There are 2 common reasons for the reappearance of wet mucus. First, a woman can identify her peak day improperly. However, the greater her experience with mucus observations, the less likely this is. Second, ovulation can be delayed. A delay in ovulation can cause wet mucus to come and go until the egg is finally released. These situations need not be a problem if 2 key points are remembered:

1. Always wait until the evening of the fourth non-wet day after the peak day to resume intercourse.
2. Always wait to resume intercourse until the thermal shift rule is applied.

The temperature pattern can greatly help you

if these situations occur since the peak day usually occurs around the same time as the thermal shift. This means that the beginning of the absolutely infertile phase is usually the same when the thermal shift and peak day rules are applied. *If the 2 rules do not coincide, the most conservative rule must be followed before resuming intercourse.*

For example, if you have applied the thermal shift rule and it gives you an absolutely infertile phase beginning Wednesday evening, yet application of the peak day rule gives an absolutely infertile phase beginning on Tuesday evening, these 2 rules do not coincide. To be sure you are no longer fertile, use the most conservative rule. In this example, intercourse should not begin on Tuesday evening but on Wednesday evening.

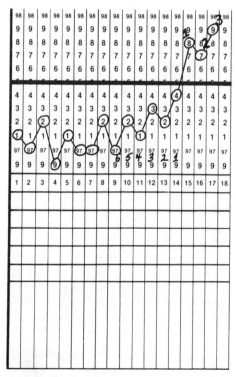

Figure 30—Use the most conservative rule

—51—

In Figure 30 — Sheri applied both the peak day rule and thermal shift rule. The peak day rule gave her an absolutely infertile phase beginning on the evening of cycle day 16. However, the thermal shift rule gave an absolutely infertile phase beginning on the evening of cycle day 17. To be safe Sheri used the most conservative rule to begin her absolutely infertile phase. In this case the thermal shift rule was followed and her absolutely infertile phase began the evening of cycle day 17.

TO REVIEW:

Use of your basal body temperature is an accurate way of determining that you have ovulated and are no longer able to become pregnant. Remember that the temperature rises after ovulation. Therefore, it makes sense to use the temperature shift in combination with the changes in cervical mucus in order to be as accurate as possible in determining the beginning of the absolutely infertile time. Another advantage in using the basal body temperature is that it can help you make sure you have identified the peak day properly.

Cervix Closing Rule for Cervical Changes

The last rule used to determine the beginning of the absolutely infertile Phase III is called the cervix closing rule. If you are checking your cervix, you will need to determine *the first day that the cervical opening begins to close.* This day is called the cervix closing day.

Remember that the cervix becomes high in the vaginal canal and soft, and the opening widens as ovulation approaches. After ovulation it moves lower in the vaginal canal becomes firm and the opening closes.

As soon as you feel the cervix lowering and firming up and the opening beginning to close, you can use the cervix closing rule.

CERVIX CLOSING RULE

The Absolutely Infertile Phase (AIP) begins on the evening of the third consecutive day of a lower, closed, and firm cervix after the cervix closing day.

By the evening of the third day, the cervix should feel low and firm, and the opening should be closed.

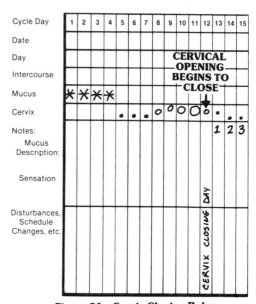

Figure 31—Cervix Closing Rule

In Figure 31 — Marie was observing her cervix and noticed that the cervical opening began to close on cycle day 12. Since it continued to close down for 3 days in a row after the cervix closing day, her absolutely infertile phase began on the evening of cycle day 15.

Caution:

If during the 3-day count the cervical opening widens, you must wait until it begins to close again and then apply the 3-day count.

Although the cervix closing rule provides you with additional information as to the beginning of the infertile time, it is not recommended that it be used alone to determine the beginning of the absolutely infertile time. When the absolutely infertile phase begins, you no longer need to check your cervix.

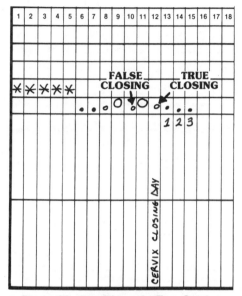

Figure 32—Identifying the True Cervix Closing Day

In Figure 32 — Julie was observing her cervix and noticed that on cycle day 10 the cervical opening felt smaller than it had the day before. She assumed this was her cervix closing day. However, on cycle day 11 the cervical opening widened again. Since she knew she either identified her cervical changes incorrectly or could be ovulating later than usual, she continued to abstain. She identified her true cervix closing day on cycle day 12. Therefore, Julie's absolutely infertile phase began on the evening of cycle day 15, the third day after the cervix began to close.

Remember:

1. When using the sympto-thermal method of natural family planning, at least the thermal shift rule and peak day rule must be used together. Using the mucus sign alone does not always enable you to tell when you have actually ovulated.

2. As we have previously mentioned, the thermal shift and peak day rules usually coincide. If the 2 rules do not coincide, *the most conservative sign should be used to determine the beginning of the absolutely infertile phase.*

A SPECIAL NOTE:

Use of natural family planning has no known physical side effects for the woman. However, there are a few studies that suggest, but do not prove, that couples who had an unplanned pregnancy using periodic abstinence had a higher incidence of spontaneous abortion as well as children born with certain mental and physical defects.

It is believed that one cause of the higher incidence of these problems is due to the fertilization of an over-ripe egg. This can occur if intercourse has not taken place before ovulation but only 1 to 2 days after the temperature rise. This can result in fertilization of an over-ripe egg.

Another possible cause of these problems is due to fertilization of an egg by an over-aged sperm. If during prolonged periods of abstinence from intercourse, ejaculation has not taken place, over-aged sperm can be present when intercourse is resumed.

We have added this information not to alarm you but to enable you to put this debatable issue into perspective. If an increase in spontaneous abortion and birth defects is related to the use of NFP, carefully following the absolutely infertile phase rules would minimize this possibility. These rules allow for the release and life span of 2 eggs. Therefore, the chances of pregnancy when intercourse is resumed are minimal.

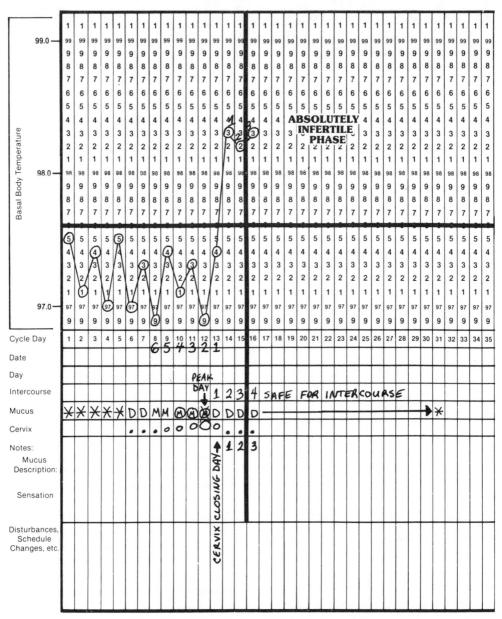

Figure 33—All the Absolutely Infertile Phase Rules

In Figure 33 — Kim observed her mucus, cervix and basal body temperature, and by applying all the rules, she saw that her absolutely infertile phase began on the evening of cycle day 16. Since her menstrual cycle was 30 days long, she could safely have intercourse from the evening of the 16th day up to and including cycle day 30. During these days she no longer needed to observe her fertility signs.

When can you begin using these rules to avoid pregnancy?

During the first cycle of observing and charting you may be able to use these rules to determine an absolutely infertile phase. However, this can be done *only* if you are certain about what you are experiencing. If you are not, you must wait at least another menstrual cycle, until you are more comfortable with your own fertility pattern, before you apply these rules. You must be confident that you are following the instructions for checking and charting properly, and applying the rules correctly, before assuming you are no longer fertile and resuming intercourse.

Using Natural Family Planning Rules to determine the before ovulation infertile Phase I

The Before Ovulation Infertile Phase I is the first phase of the menstrual cycle. It begins with the first day of menstrual bleeding. It is the period of days before ovulation when intercourse can take place with a very small chance of pregnancy. To determine the length of this phase, the Alternate Dry Day Rule is applied.

Alternate Dry Day

After the end of menstrual bleeding, if mucus appears, the fertile phase begins. If it does not appear, the Alternate Dry Day Rule can be used to provide safe days for intercourse before ovulation.

The Alternate Dry Day Rule states that intercourse can take place the evening of every other dry day. A dry day is a complete day of no mucus and dry vaginal sensation. Once intercourse occurs, semen can prevent the

accurate observation of mucus for up to 24 hours. Because of this there is no way of telling if the secretions from the vagina are semen, mucus, or perhaps a combination of both. Since this rule is used to detect early-warning mucus, abstinence must be followed for one full day, after which time the semen will be gone and observing mucus is once again possible. If the day following a full day of abstinence is dry again, intercourse can be resumed on the evening of that day.

ALTERNATE DRY DAY RULE

Once the menstrual bleeding ends, intercourse can take place the evening of every other dry day.

Some women have found that urinating and using the Kegel Exercise right after intercourse pushes all the semen out of the vagina, making the day after intercourse dry. If this works for you, there is no reason to abstain on that day and intercourse can occur on that evening. In other words, if you are dry the entire day after intercourse, you do not have to follow the Alternate Dry Day Rule.

Some women are comfortable having intercourse during menstruation and would like to know if intercourse during this time can lead to pregnancy. The chance of pregnancy is slim if the True Menses Rule is followed.

True Menses Rule

The True Menses Rule states that the first 4 days of the menstrual cycle are safe for intercourse with a 99% to 99.9% effectiveness rate in avoiding pregnancy. In order to use the first 4 days for intercourse, 2 conditions must be met. First, the woman has to have experienced a thermal shift during the previous cycle. This proves that ovulation has occurred and the bleeding she has is true menstrual bleeding. Second, the last 6 cycles need to have lasted 25 days or longer.

TRUE MENSES RULE

The first 4 days of the menstrual cycle are safe for intercourse if ovulation took place in the previous cycle and the most recent 6 cycles were at least 25 days in length.

Only the first 4 days of the menstrual cycle are 99% to 99.9% safe for intercourse. This means that if a woman's menstrual bleeding lasts for 3 days, the first 4 days are safe for intercourse. For those women who are comfortable having intercourse during their menstrual bleeding, this rule provides days early in the cycle when the possibility of pregnancy is extremely low.

TO REVIEW:

1. *The Alternate Dry Day Rule is as the name implies. Intercourse can safely occur the evening of every other dry day before the time of ovulation nears. If intercourse takes place, abstaining the next day allows the semen to leave the vaginal area. (The only time you don't have to abstain the day after intercourse is when you are dry the entire day.)*
2. *Using the first 4 days of the menstrual cycle for intercourse by applying the True Menses Rule provides additional safe days early in the cycle. IF A WOMAN CAN'T PROVE THAT HER MENSTRUAL BLEEDING IS TRUE MENSTRUAL BLEEDING BY HAVING A THERMAL SHIFT THE PREVIOUS CYCLE, SHE SHOULD CONSIDER DAYS OF BLEEDING AS FERTILE DAYS AND FOLLOW ABSTINENCE.*

The Alternate Dry Day Rule is an excellent rule for those women who wish to observe their mucus. By using this rule, women can know when to have intercourse safely before the egg is released and before the fertile mucus is around to keep sperm alive. However, some women ask, "Is there another way I can know when my fertile time is going to begin, whether or not I am observing mucus?" There is a way! For those women who do not want to observe mucus or who want to know in advance when their fertile phase is going to begin, they can use the Calculated Infertile Phase Rule. This rule got its name because it is a simple mathematical formula that gives the length of the infertile time before ovulation.

This is how to apply the rule: Find the shortest menstrual cycle that you have had in the last 6 cycles. You do not need to have kept a record of your fertility signs for these 6 cycles. You need to know only when the cycles began in order to use this rule. Subtract 21 from your shortest cycle. By doing this you will have the number of days in your calculated infertile phase (or before ovulation infertile time).

For example, let's say Susan marks on her calendar when she began menstruating for the last 6 cycles. She finds that her cycles varied from 29 to 32 days in length. The shortest cycle was 29 days. She then subtracts 21 from 29. The number left after subtracting 21 from 29 is 8 ($29 - 21 = 8$). Therefore, Susan's calculated infertile phase I is 8 days long. She can have intercourse from the first day of her menstrual cycle up to and including the eighth day of her cycle with a minimum chance of pregnancy.

CALCULATED INFERTILE PHASE RULE

The Calculated Infertile Phase (CIP) begins on the first day of menstruation. Its length is found by subtracting 21 from the shortest of the 6 most recent and consecutive normal menstrual cycles. These menstrual cycles must be at least 25 days in length.

In another example, Ann's menstrual cycles during the months of December through May (6 cycles) were 28 to 30 days long. If she subtracts 21 from the shortest of these cycles, she has a calculated infertile phase of 7 days. Since her shortest cycle was 28 days in length, Ann has the first 7 days $(28 - 21 = 7)$ of her menstrual cycle to have intercourse.

The fertile phase begins the day after the calculated infertile phase ends. In Ann's case, since the calculated infertile phase ended on day 7, her fertile phase began on day 8. Her fertile phase will continue until she can successfully apply the thermal shift and peak day rules.

Why is the number 21 used to determine the length of the calculated infertile phase? Usually the greatest number of days that occur from ovulation to the end of the cycle is 16. The longest time that sperm can survive in fertile mucus is 5 days. Of course, $16 + 5 = 21$. Subtracting 21 from the shortest menstrual cycle gives the number of days that are very safe for intercourse during the early part of the menstrual cycle.

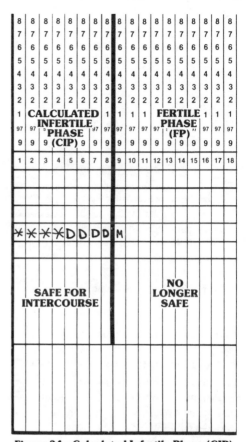

Figure 34—Calculated Infertile Phase (CIP)

In Figure 34 — Margo's previous 6 menstrual cycles have varied from 29 to 33 days in length. By subtracting 21 from 29 she had a calculated infertile phase of 8 days. She can have intercourse from the first day of the menstrual cycle up to and including cycle day 8 with a minimal chance of pregnancy. Since her calculated infertile phase ends on cycle day 8, her fertile phase begins on cycle day 9. She would then abstain until her absolutely infertile phase begins.

Remember, use this rule only if:

1. You can recall accurately when your last 6 cycles began

—or—

2. You have kept a record of the beginning of your last 6 cycles

—or—

3. You have been charting your fertility signs for 6 cycles.

To use the Calculated Infertile Phase Rule, follow these requirements carefully:
1. Use the most recent 6 cycles.
2. They must be normal cycles (for example, not birth control pill cycles, and they should be within the normal range of 25 to 37 days long).

An important factor in using this rule is the use of the most recent 6 cycles to determine the calculated infertile phase. For example, if for 6 cycles you never experienced a menstrual cycle shorter than 30 days in length, but then your seventh menstrual cycle was 28 days long, you must change your calculated infertile phase. When your cycles are 30 days long, your calculated infertile phase was 9 days in length $(30 - 21 = 9)$. However, now that you have had a 28-day menstrual cycle, your calculated infertile phase would be 7 days long. The length of a woman's menstrual cycles can normally vary a few days. If this happens to you, always make sure you use the shortest of the 6 most recent menstrual cycles to determine your calculated infertile phase.

The use of the rule is 95% to 99% effective in avoiding pregnancy. The small 1% to 5% pregnancy rate is due to the fact that the rule does not take into account an unexpected early ovulation. The warning sign of an early ovulation is cervical mucus. If the woman is having intercourse during her calculated infertile phase, semen is present in the vagina. Therefore, she may not be able to see the warning mucus. If she continues to have intercourse and ovulates earlier than usual, pregnancy can occur.

For example, Joan's menstrual cycles for the past 2 years have been 30 to 32 days long. Her calculated infertile phase is 9 days long $(30 - 21 = 9)$. For the first 9 days of her cycle, Joan has had intercourse whenever she desired and has not become pregnant. In one menstrual cycle Joan ovulated early. She was not aware of it because she was not watching her mucus sign, which would have been the signal for the early ovulation. She continued to have intercourse when mucus was present and became pregnant.

Is there a way of decreasing the chance of pregnancy during the calculated infertile phase? There is if the Alternate Dry Day Rule is followed. When a woman can calculate the length of her before-ovulation time by using the Calculated Infertile Phase Rule, she also has the choice of using the Alternate Dry Day Rule, which will enable her to see her body signaling her that her ovulation is going to happen earlier than usual. The early-warning mucus is that body signal. The woman can also choose to abstain during menstrual bleeding or use the True Menses Rule. It all depends upon the effectiveness rate she wants.

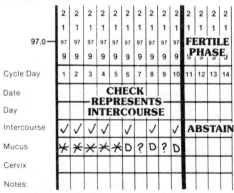

Figure 35—The Calculated Infertile Phase (CIP) Rule, True Menses Rule, and Alternate Dry Day Rule

In Figure 35 — Naomi's calculated infertile phase is 10 days long. Because she would like to have a 99 to 99.9% effective time to have intercourse before ovulating, she used the true menses rule and alternate dry day rule during her calculated infertile phase. By applying the true menses rule, the first 4 days were safe for intercourse. Since she was still bleeding on cycle day 5, she could not observe possible mucus. On cycle day 6 she experienced a dry day. By using the alternate dry day rule, she had intercourse on the evening of that day. She abstained throughout cycle day 7 to allow semen to leave the vaginal area. On cycle day 8 she continued to abstain until she was sure the entire day was dry again. Because it was, she had intercourse on that evening. She abstained on cycle day 9 again and because cycle day 10 was dry the entire day, it was still safe for intercourse. Since her calculated infertile phase ended on day 10, her fertile phase began on day 11. On cycle day 11 she began her period of abstinence.

Caution:

If any mucus is detected within the calculated infertile phase, the woman must consider herself potentially fertile since the mucus may indicate an early ovulation.

Fertile Phase II

We have described how to determine the beginning and the end of the calculated infertile Phase I and how to determine the beginning and the end of the absolutely infertile Phase III. The fertile Phase II is the number of days between Phase I and Phase III. It begins the day after the calculated infertile Phase I ends or the first day any mucus appears, whichever comes first.

For example, Ann's calculated infertile phase is 9 days long. She is using the alternate dry day rule and notices mucus on day 7. Since this mucus could be an indication of an early ovulation, her calculated infertile phase would end earlier than usual and day 7 would begin her fertile phase.

It is during the fertile phase that the possibility of pregnancy is greatest. **Therefore, intercourse and genital to genital contact must be avoided if pregnancy is not desired.** The fertile phase ends when the absolutely infertile phase rules have been applied.

Summary of the 3 Phases of the Menstrual Cycle

Phase I, the Calculated Infertile Phase, includes:

1. The menstrual flow.
2. Days which are dry (mucus is not present and there is a dry vaginal sensation).
3. Days in which the cervix is low, firm and closed.
4. Low basal body temperatures, with the possible exception of a few higher temperatures which may occur during the menstrual flow.

Phase II, the Fertile Phase, includes:

1. All mucus days until the peak day rule is applied.
2. Days in which the cervix is higher in the vaginal canal, soft and open until the cervix closing rule is applied (optional rule).
3. The rising of the basal body temperature from low pre-ovulatory levels to high post-ovulatory levels until the thermal shift rule is applied.

Phase III, the Absolutely Infertile Phase, includes:

1. Days when mucus is of a non-wet quality and/or days which are completely dry, and it may include a few wet days at the end of the menstrual cycle.

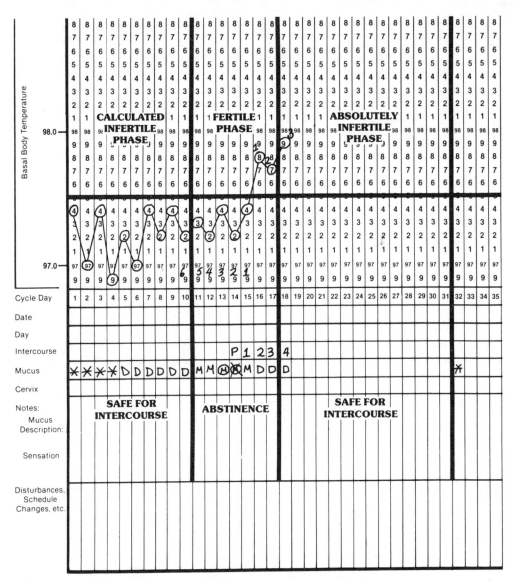

Figure 36—The Three Phases of the Menstrual Cycle

In Figure 36 — Angela's last 6 menstrual cycles were 31 days in length. Therefore, her calculated infertile phase is 10 days long. Depending upon the effectiveness rate she chooses, she can have intercourse whenever she desires during the calculated infertile phase or use the true menses rule, alternate dry day rule or both during the calculated infertile phase. Her fertile phase began on cycle day 11.

Abstinence was observed until the absolutely infertile phase rules could be applied. She chose to observe her mucus and basal body temperatures but not her cervix. By application of the thermal shift rule and peak day rule, she could resume intercourse on the evening of cycle day 18 up to and including cycle day 31.

2. Days in which the cervix is low, firm, and closed.
3. Days in which the temperature remains in the high post-ovulatory levels for about 12 to 16 days.

Short Cycle Calculations

We stated that if a woman wants to safely have intercourse before ovulation takes place, the menstrual cycles must be 25 days or longer. This means that *women who have cycles shorter than 25 days begin their fertile phase on the first day of the menstrual cycle.*

Short cycles mean that ovulation takes place early in the cycle, a few days after the menstrual flow ends. Because of this, cervical mucus can be present during the menstrual flow. The bleeding makes observation of the mucus difficult if not impossible. If intercourse occurs and mucus is present, the sperm may be able to survive long enough to fertilize the egg at ovulation. The result is that for a woman with short cycles, pregnancy may occur from intercourse taking place during the first few days of her menstrual cycle.

Therefore, a woman with short cycles has 2 instead of 3 phases to her menstrual cycle, a

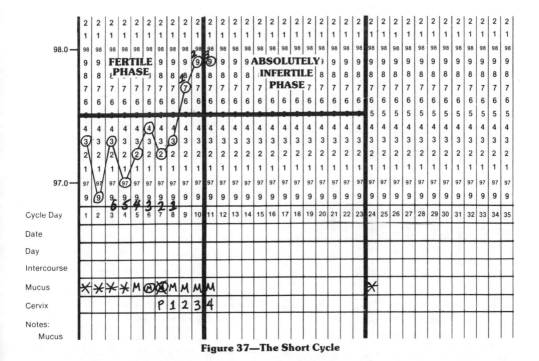

Figure 37—The Short Cycle

In Figure 37 — Jade's previous 6 menstrual cycles were 23 to 26 days in length. Since she normally experiences short menstrual cycles, she does not have a calculated infertile phase. Therefore, her fertile phase begins on the first day of her menstrual cycle and ends when she can successfully apply the abso-

lutely infertile phase rules. In this example she had to abstain from cycle day 1 through cycle day 11. She could resume intercourse the evening of cycle day 11 up to and including the end of her menstrual cycle, day 23.

fertile and an absolutely infertile phase. *The first day of menstrual bleeding is the first day of the fertile phase. The fertile phase ends and the absolutely infertile phase begins when the thermal shift rule and peak day rule have been applied.*

The Basic Infertile Pattern

There are a few women who always have the *same type* of mucus as soon as the menstrual flow ends. These women experience the same type of mucus every day during the calculated infertile phase. This situation of daily non-changing mucus is called a basic infertile mucus pattern. Since there are no dry days during the calculated infertile phase, the alternate dry day rule is applied to the non-changing mucus. In other words, the non-changing mucus days are used as though they were dry, no-mucus days. Therefore, *intercourse may occur the evening of every other non-changing mucus day.*

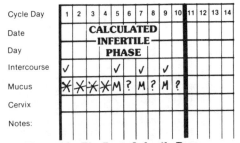

Figure 38—The Basic Infertile Pattern

In Figure 38 — Cheryl had observed the same type of mucus every day during her calculated infertile phase of 10 days. Because she felt she had gained the experience to be confident with her mucus observations, she used the days of non-changing mucus (or her basic infertile pattern) as though they were dry days. In other words, Cheryl had 2 choices — to use any day of the calculated infertile phase to have intercourse, or to increase the level of effectiveness in this phase by following the true menses rule, alternate dry day rule or both. This example illustrates her use of the alternate dry day rule and the true menses rule.

These women must be careful to be on the lookout for any change in their basic infertile patterns. *If the mucus changes in any way, it may mean that ovulation is approaching.* If the mucus does change, the fertile phase has started and abstinence must begin.

Caution:

A woman may need to observe the mucus for 2 or more menstrual cycles to develop the experience necessary to use this rule.

A SPECIAL NOTE ABOUT CERVICAL MUCUS:

It is important to remember that certain factors can affect the cervical mucus, preventing the accurate observations needed to successfully apply the mucus rules.

These factors are:

1. **Douching**, which removes most cervical mucus from the vaginal canal. (It does not remove all of it, which is why douching is not a successful method of birth control. However, it can remove enough of the mucus to make cervical mucus observations inaccurate.)

2. **Semen**, which is left in the vaginal canal after intercourse. It mixes with cervical mucus making the observation of the mucus very difficult if not impossible.

3. **Sexual arousal**, which causes moisture to form in the vaginal canal, can make it difficult to determine when mucus is present. You should wait until the wet feeling from sexual arousal is gone before checking for cervical mucus.

4. **Spermicidal agents** (creams, jellies and foams), which remain in the vagina for a day or more after their use. You should not use them if you want to

observe your mucus as accurately as possible.

5. **A vaginal infection** will prevent accurate observation of cervical mucus. The way to handle this situation is discussed further in Chapter 10.

If you wish to use all the natural family planning rules well, it is important to do the following:

1. **Observe your fertility signs accurately.**
2. **Chart your fertility signs and changes accurately.**
3. **Follow the rules as they have been explained.**

One More Situation to Think About

What should a woman do if she does not have an accurate history of her most recent 6 menstrual cycles or has just stopped using birth control pills? In both of these situations she does not have the proper information to use the Calculated Infertile Phase Rule. To be most conservative and safe, the woman should consider herself fertile from the first day of menstrual bleeding until her absolutely infertile phase begins. Once she has 6 cycles recorded, the calculated infertile phase rule can be used to determine the safe days early in the menstrual cycle.

However, some women find that waiting for 6 cycles to pass is unsatisfactory. They would like to have intercourse safely before ovulation even though they are not able to use the CIP rule. These women choose to use the Alternate Dry Day Rule. In other words, they abstain during menstrual bleeding and once the bleeding ends, they begin observing their cervical mucus. If mucus is not present throughout the entire day and dry vaginal sensations are experienced, they can have intercourse in the evening of the dry day. They then continue to use the Alternate Dry Day Rule until mucus production begins. (See page 58 for review of this rule.) Once mucus is observed and/or the vaginal sensations are no longer dry, the fertile phase has begun. Abstinence would be followed until the start of the absolutely infertile phase.

notes:

CHAPTER X

THE EARLY YEARS, THE LATER YEARS, BREAST FEEDING, ILLNESSES, ETC.
Special Circumstances

It is not uncommon for us to make plans which have to be changed at the last minute. Yet, the change need not "ruin our day" if we allow room for it to happen.

This is true of the fertility cycle. Natural family planning can be used successfully with the normal ovulatory cycle, and if something happens to cause a change in the cycle or the patterns of the fertility signs, they can still be followed to avoid pregnancy.

Any situations which cause a change in your menstrual cycle or patterns of fertility signs are called special circumstances.

If a special circumstance occurs, you can usually continue to use fertility signs successfully to avoid pregnancy. Pregnancy can be avoided by knowing what to look for and by using the special circumstances rules explained in this chapter.

Special circumstances include:

> *Fever*
> *Breastfeeding*
> *Stress*
> *Ovarian cyst*
> *Birth control pills*
> *Exercise*
> *Diet*
> *Travel*
> *Illness*
> *Premenopause*

The most frequent special circumstances are the common illnesses. The most common of these are the cold and flu. These are types of infections that can cause the body temperature to rise unusually high. This is known as a fever. When you have a fever, your basal body temperature will remain high until you begin to recover from the illness.

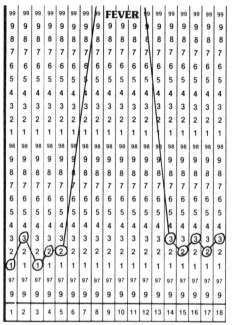

Figure 39—Charting a fever

In Figure 39 — Sue began observing and recording her basal body temperature from the first day of her menstrual cycle. From cycle day 6 through cycle day 13 she experienced a fever above 99.1 degrees. She noted the presence of a fever on her chart. When the fever subsided, she resumed observing and recording her basal body temperature.

Having a fever need not be a difficult or confusing situation if you are using basal body temperature to avoid pregnancy. If you see your temperature rising higher than usual or rising earlier than expected (whether or not you are feeling ill), you need to watch this unexpected temperature change carefully. If a fever is present, your temperature should be taken with a fever thermometer once in the morning and once in the evening until the fever is no longer present. A fever ther-

mometer should be used since it measures the body temperature up to 108 degrees. The basal body thermometer only goes up to 100 degrees. You will not be able to know how high your fever actually is if you use your basal body thermometer. It could also break if it is used to try to measure unusually high temperatures.

The unusually high temperature should be recorded on the fertility awareness chart in a special way each day it is present. If the temperature is higher than the temperatures printed on the chart (the chart goes up to 99 degrees), a line should be drawn from the last normal basal body temperature to the very top of the chart. Each day the temperature remains off the chart, it should be recorded in the notes column. When you begin to recover from the illness, the basal body temperature will return to a normal level. You should then resume taking your temperature with the basal body thermometer and recording it as usual.

When you have an illness that causes a fever, one of 3 situations may occur during the menstrual cycle:

1. Ovulation will occur as usual and the menstrual cycle will be its usual length.
2. Ovulation will occur later than usual and the menstrual cycle will be longer than its usual length.
3. Ovulation will not occur and an unusual bleeding pattern may be seen. Even if this bleeding takes place around the time you would expect to see menstrual bleeding, do not consider this true menstrual bleeding.

Ovulation on Time

When the high temperature from illness occurs

during the time of ovulation, a thermal shift cannot be seen. However, you will know if you ovulate because once the fever is gone, the temperature will drop back down to the high temperatures you normally experience after ovulation.

Observe your mucus and cervical changes during the fever. However, even if the peak day rule can be applied, you should still wait until the thermal shift rule can also be applied to be sure ovulation has taken place and the absolutely infertile phase has begun.

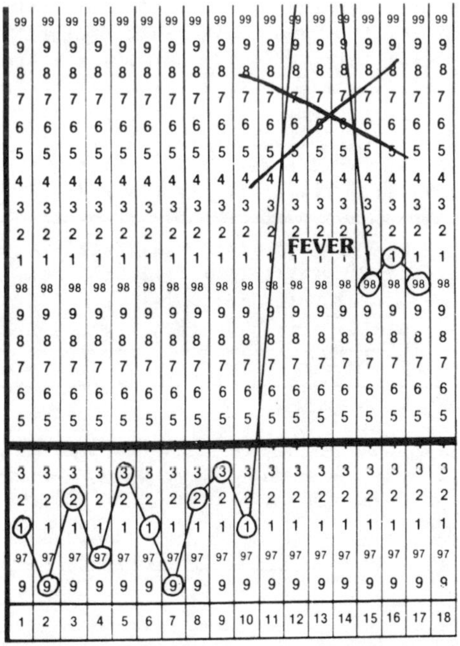

Figure 40—Fever during time of ovulation

In Figure 40 — Alice experienced a fever from cycle day 11 through cycle day 15. Once the fever subsided, her basal body temperature was at the normal post-ovulatory levels. This indicated that ovulation had taken place at some point during the fever. To determine the absolutely infertile phase, she drew a coverline above the highest of the 6 normal low pre-ovulatory temperatures recorded before the fever.

Late Ovulation

Ovulation may be delayed during an illness. A delayed ovulation is one that happens later than usual during the menstrual cycle. With a delayed ovulation the thermal shift may not be seen until a few days to a week later than usual. If ovulation did not occur during the fever, the temperatures will return to their normal low pre-ovulatory levels once the fever has subsided. Again, the thermal shift rule and peak day rule should be applied to be sure ovulation has taken place and the absolutely infertile phase has begun.

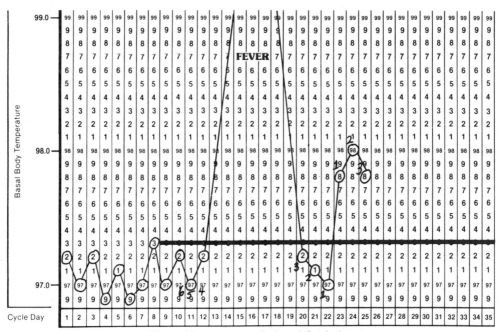

Figure 41—Fever and Delayed Ovulation

In Figure 41 — Elisa usually has menstrual cycles ranging from 28 to 32 days in length. During a cycle when she was ill, she experienced ovulation later than what was usual for her. This was seen by the fact that when her fever subsided on cycle day 20, her basal body temperature was still low. On cycle day 23 her temperature shifted and she was then able to apply the thermal shift rule to determine her absolutely infertile phase.

No Ovulation

No ovulation is called **anovulation.** *You may not ovulate at all during the time of illness.*

Basal Body Temperature Patterns During the Anovulatory Cycle

When ovulation does not occur, you will continue to experience a low temperature pattern. This low pattern is just like the one you normally see before ovulation. The thermal shift does not occur. In other words, since ovulation has not taken place, you are unable to apply the thermal shift rule. However, you will be able to use your mucus observations, with special rules discussed later in this chapter, to avoid pregnancy.

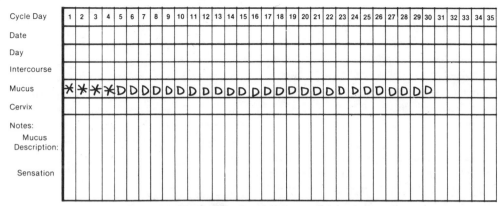

Cycle Day	1	2	3	4	5	6	7	8	9	10	11	12	13	14	15	16	17	18	19	20	21	22	23	24	25	26	27	28	29	30	31	32	33	34	35
Date																																			
Day																																			
Intercourse																																			
Mucus	✳	✳	✳	✳	D	D	D	D	D	D	D	D	D	D	D	D	D	D	D	D	D	D	D	D	D	D	D	D	D	D	D				
Cervix																																			
Notes: Mucus Description:																																			
Sensation																																			

Figure 42 —Anovulation and no mucus

In Figure 42 — Jeanine had the flu one cycle, causing a time of anovulation. During the entire time she did not ovulate, mucus was not produced and a continuous dry vaginal sensation was present.

Cervical Mucus Patterns During the Anovulatory Cycle

When ovulation does not occur, there is no one special pattern of mucus.

- You may produce mucus that remains sticky, pasty and dry throughout the entire time you do not ovulate.
- You may not produce any mucus and remain dry at the outside of your vaginal area.
- You may experience wet mucus and a wet feeling at the outside of your vaginal area. The mucus may be of the creamy, wet type or may even feel somewhat slippery and stretchy. However, the mucus will not become the very wet, stretchy and slippery type that occurs with ovulation.
- You may experience a combination of these changes. For example, you may have dry days and sticky, pasty, non-wet mucus days during the entire time you do not ovulate. Or

you may experience non-wet mucus days, totally dry days and wet days during the entire time you do not ovulate.

Cervical Changes During the Anovulatory Cycle

- You may experience a low, firm and closed cervix while you are not ovulating.
- You may experience a slightly raised, slightly soft and slightly open cervix while you are not ovulating.
- You may even experience a combination of both, low to slightly high, firm to slightly soft and closed to slightly open.

If you do not ovulate, you may or may not bleed, or spotting of blood may occur. If you do experience bleeding, it may be lighter or heavier than normal, and it may last a shorter or longer period of time than your usual menstrual bleeding. The important thing to remember is that *if bleeding of any type occurs during the times of anovulation, it is not menstrual bleeding. It could be a warning that ovulation is taking place or is going to take place. Therefore, any bleeding is treated as though it is mucus. It is a fertile time!*

We have given several possibilities for changes in fertility signs during the anovulatory cycle because a woman can experience a range of changes during times of anovulation.

A word of comfort — if you observe your signs carefully, you can know what is happening to you!

Secondary Signs and Premenstrual Signs

If you usually experience bodily changes which alert you to the approach of ovulation and your menstrual flow, they may be different or you may not experience them at all during the time that ovulation does not occur.

Temporary infertility means that fertility can return at any time. Since there isn't a way to predict when ovulation will return, the following special circumstances rules must be followed carefully when you question whether or not you are experiencing either delayed ovulation or anovulation. Since these rules will allow you to be on the lookout for signs of returning fertility, they will protect you against pregnancy.

Special Circumstances Rules

These rules are applied to the mucus observations when experiencing anovulation or delayed ovulation. *If properly followed, they can enable a woman to have intercourse safely while still being able to observe any mucus changes that could mean ovulation is approaching and therefore a return of fertility.*

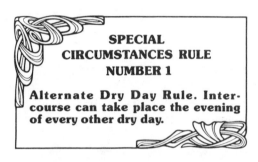

SPECIAL CIRCUMSTANCES RULE NUMBER 1

Alternate Dry Day Rule. Intercourse can take place the evening of every other dry day.

1. Alternate Dry Day Rule

As you may recall, this rule states that intercourse may safely occur on the evening of every other dry day. A dry day means a day of no mucus and a dry vaginal sensation. The day after intercourse must be an abstinence day. If semen is present in the vagina the day after intercourse, you will not know if mucus is present and if ovulation is going to take place. Intercourse can continue every other dry day throughout the time of anovulation.

Anovulation = No Ovulation = A Time of Temporary Infertility

Cycle Day	1	2	3	4	5	6	7	8	9	10	11	12	13	14	15	16	17	18	19	20	21	22	23	24	25	26	27	28	29	30	31	32	33	34	35
Date																																			
Day																																			
Intercourse	√		√				√				√		√				√				√				√		√						√		√
Mucus	D	?	D	?	D	D	D	D	D	D	?	D	?	D	D	D	D	D	?	D	D	D	?	D	D	D	?	D	?	D	D	D	D	?	D
Cervix																																			

Figure 43—Use of the Alternate Dry Day Rule and Anovulation

In Figure 43 — Diane has not ovulated for 2 months. Because she has experienced continuous dry days, she has used the alternate dry day rule whenever she has had intercourse.

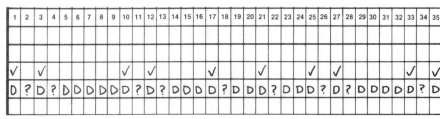

SPECIAL CIRCUMSTANCE RULE NUMBER 2

Mucus Patch Rule. Abstinence from intercourse should be followed if one or more days of any type of mucus occurs after a dry day

AND

if the mucus is of a non-wet quality with a dry vaginal sensation, abstinence should be followed for 2 dry days after the mucus is no longer present

OR

if the mucus is of a wet quality with a wet vaginal sensation, abstinence should be followed for 4 dry days after the mucus is no longer present

2. Mucus Patch Rule

This rule states that if, following a dry day, you experience one day or more of any type of mucus, you must abstain from intercourse. This mucus could mean that ovulation is approaching.

If the mucus is the sticky, non-wet mucus and a dry vaginal sensation is present, you need to abstain during those days when the mucus is present and for 2 dry days after the non-wet mucus ends. Then you can resume applying the alternate dry day rule.

If the mucus is the wet-feeling mucus and a wet vaginal sensation is present, you need to abstain during those days when the mucus is present and for 4 dry days after the wet-feeling mucus ends. Then you can resume applying the alternate dry day rule.

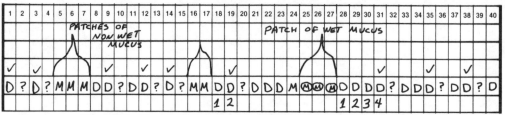

Figure 44—Use of the Alternate Dry Day Rule and Mucus Patch Rule during Anovulation

In Figure 44 — Morgan has been using the alternate dry day rule during the past 35 days. One day while checking for mucus, she notices the presence of sticky, non-wet mucus. Since this could be a sign of approaching ovulation, she begins to abstain. She finds that she has 3 days of the non-wet mucus and then returns to experiencing completely dry days. In this situation, Morgan abstains during the 3 days of mucus and for 2 dry days after the mucus ends. Because she did not ovulate, she resumes using the alternate dry day rule until mucus is again produced.

Morgan continues to use the alternate dry day rule for dry days and the mucus patch rule for non-wet mucus days. One day she notices a wet vaginal sensation and observes wet-feeling mucus. Since ovulation may be near, she abstains during the time when mucus is present. Once the mucus ends, she continues to abstain for 4 dry days instead of 2 dry days. This is because the mucus is wet. After applying the mucus patch rule, she can resume using the alternate dry day rule during her completely dry days.

TO REVIEW:

1. *Intercourse can occur the evening of every other dry day.*
2. *Abstinence should be followed during any days of mucus. If the mucus is non-wet, abstinence continues until the evening of the second dry day after the non-wet mucus ends. If the mucus is wet, abstinence continues until the evening of the fourth dry day after the wet mucus ends.*

The Basic Infertile Pattern of Cervical Mucus

During the times when a woman is not ovulating she may experience what is called a basic infertile pattern of cervical mucus. This means that instead of experiencing mostly dry days, *she experiences the same type of cervical mucus every day.* Usually this non-changing mucus is the dry-feeling, pasty, sticky, non-wet type or the slightly creamy type of mucus.

If this occurs, the non-changing mucus days are treated as though they were dry days. In other words, you can have intercourse every other non-changing mucus day. However, if you experience any change in the basic infertile pattern, you need to abstain because you may be approaching ovulation. To prevent pregnancy in this situation, the mucus patch rule should be used. *The mucus patch rule for the basic infertile mucus pattern states that abstinence should begin as soon as there is any change in the quality of the basic infertile mucus. Abstinence should continue throughout the changing mucus and for 4 days after it ends.* If it does not become the very wet, stretchy, slippery mucus of ovulation and/or the thermal shift rule cannot be applied, then ovulation probably did not occur. In this situation, intercourse can be resumed after the mucus has returned to the basic infertile mucus pattern for 4 days in a row. Then the alternate dry day rule is used until another mucus patch is observed.

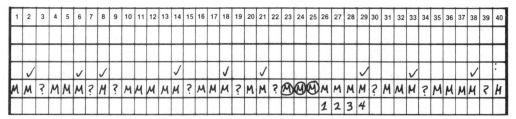

Figure 45 —Use of the Alternate Dry Day Rule and Mucus Patch Rule with a basic infertile mucus pattern

In Figure 45 — Marlene has been experiencing anovulation for 3 months. During this time she has observed the same kind of mucus day after day. So she has been using the alternate dry day rule. One day she notices the mucus has changed. It feels and looks different. This could be a sign of the approach of ovulation. Because of this she abstains during the days of the different mucus. As soon as the mucus has returned to its basic infertile pattern for 4 days in a row, she can resume using the alternate dry day rule.

TO REVIEW:

1. Intercourse can occur the evening of every other non-changing mucus day (alternate dry day rule).
2. If the mucus changes, the mucus patch rule is applied.
3. Once the mucus patch rule has been applied, the alternate dry day rule can again be used.
4. Abstinence should be followed during any days of changing mucus.

If any type of bleeding occurs during a time of anovulation, these days are treated as though they are wet mucus days. Bleeding can mean ovulation. Therefore, abstinence should be followed during any days of bleeding and for 4 dry days after the bleeding ends. If ovulation takes place during bleeding, you will see a thermal shift at this time. However, bleeding makes it difficult to observe mucus accurately.

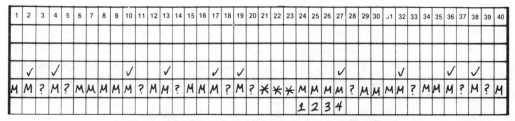

Figure 46—Anovulation Mucus Patch and bleeding

In Figure 46 — during the fourth month of anovulation, Marlene experiences bleeding. Since this could mean ovulation is occurring, she abstains during the bleeding. As soon as the mucus has returned to its basic infertile pattern for 4 days after the bleeding ends, she can resume using the alternate dry day rule.

Although anovulation lasts for a varied period of time, ovulation will usually return. When it does return, you will observe the thermal shift and the very wet, slippery, stretchy mucus, as well as the other usual ovulatory mucus changes. The thermal shift rule and peak day rule can then be applied to determine the absolutely infertile phase.

Once ovulation returns, you should observe 6 ovulatory cycles in a row before you use the calculated infertile phase rule (with or without the true menses and alternate dry day rules). Remember that the menstrual cycles may change after a period of anovulation. Therefore, it is important to observe 6 cycles before applying the calculated infertile phase rule.

Anovulation has many causes. An illness with a fever is just one example. Some other causes of anovulation include:

• Illness
Some women's reproductive systems are greatly affected by any type of illness. Ovulation can stop because of an illness but will usually return once the illness is over.

• Birth Control Pills
Birth control pills work to prevent pregnancy primarily by stopping ovulation. Once you stop taking them, ovulation may begin within 2 to 3 weeks or may not begin for a month or more. Even if ovulation begins right away and a thermal shift is observed, it may take a month or more for the mucus to return to a normal ovulatory mucus pattern. In other words, some women see a thermal shift, but the mucus does not seem to become the very wet, slippery, stretchy mucus. Because of this, the peak day rule cannot be applied. If this occurs, the thermal shift rule can be used alone with a minimal possibility of pregnancy.

• Change in Diet and/or Exercise Routine
When a woman changes her eating habits and/or exercise routine, she usually experiences a change in her body weight. Sometimes a 5 to 10-pound weight gain or loss can cause a change in the ovulatory pattern or can cause anovulation. A change in diet and/or exercise without a weight loss or gain can also have the same effect. Once the body becomes adjusted to this change in weight, ovulation usually returns.

• Menopause
As a woman approaches her late 30's to her 40's, she will usually experience gradual changes in her menstrual cycle. She may not ovulate every month, ovulate every 2 to 3 months or even less frequently. After one full year of no menstrual bleeding, the possibility of ovulating is small. Once the full year has passed, a woman has reached the menopausal period of her life. Since a woman approaching menopause may ovulate infrequently, she should use the alternate dry day and mucus patch rules during the times of anovulation. When she does ovulate, she can apply the thermal shift and peak day rules to determine the absolutely infertile phase. A woman ovulating infrequently cannot use the calculated infertile phase rule. Therefore, the days of menstrual bleeding following ovulation would be considered fertile. Once the bleeding ends, she can resume the use of the alternate dry day rule and mucus patch rule until she ovulates and the absolutely infertile phase rules can be applied.

• Emotional Stress
The way you feel emotionally can affect your body physically. Over the past few years the relationship of the mind and body has

been studied to a great extent. It is well known that emotional stress can cause ulcers, backaches and headaches. All of us experience stressful events in our lives: changing jobs, a death in the family, travel, family visits, and on and on. Any of these may cause you not to ovulate for a month or more.

• Development of an Ovarian Cyst
Occasionally the developing follicle may not continue to the point of ovulation. Instead it enlarges to form a cyst on the ovary, lasting about 2 to 6 weeks. Usually ovulation does not occur while the cyst is present. During this time irregular bleeding may be experienced or the menstrual period can be delayed a week or more.

Again, as with all other causes of delayed ovulation and anovulation, the alternate dry day rule and mucus patch rule are used.

• Breastfeeding
During the time of breastfeeding ovulation may occur irregularly or not at all. This usually depends upon the way you choose to breastfeed.

If you breastfeed throughout the day, each and every time the baby is hungry or when the baby just desires the comfort of suckling the mother's breast, there is a small chance of ovulation. This is because that small gland at the base of the brain, the pituitary gland, produces a hormone that stops ovulation. The amount of the hormone produced depends upon the number of times a day the baby is breastfed.

If you give the baby water, juice or other types of nourishment, as well as allowing the baby to suck on a pacifier, you have a greater chance of ovulating. In this case it is important to always observe your fertility signs carefully. This is especially true when you stop feeding the baby at night or if anything else occurs which leads to the baby suckling the breast less often.

The decision of how and why to breastfeed will depend upon many factors, including whether you are working or involved in other activities which prevent you from being with the baby throughout the day. Unfortunately, some women have been told that if they breastfeed once or twice a day, they will not ovulate and cannot become pregnant. This is not true. The return of ovulation is affected by the amount of suckling that occurs throughout the day. The less often each day the baby has an opportunity to suckle the breast, the greater the chance of ovulation.

The return of ovulation, and therefore fertility, will vary from woman to woman. In general, the earliest return of ovulation for a woman who is totally breastfeeding is about 10 weeks after delivery. The average return of ovulation for a woman who is totally breastfeeding is about 14½ months after delivery. When bottle feeding the baby, ovulation can begin within 2 to 4 weeks after delivery. The return of ovulation will depend partially upon when supplementary feeding is introduced, as well as when and how weaning of the baby begins. When fertility returns, the clear slippery mucus with a true wet vaginal sensation, the shift in temperature, and a high, soft and open cervix will be observed.

In general, a woman who is breastfeeding may experience one or more of these mucus patterns:

1. She may be completely dry, with no mucus during the entire time of total breastfeeding.

2. She may experience one day or more of non-wet, pasty, sticky mucus between dry days.
3. Occasionally a totally breastfeeding woman may also experience wet sensations and wet mucus, usually of the more creamy type. This type of mucus can be present between dry days or days of non-wet, pasty, sticky mucus.
4. After the weaning process begins, a woman is apt to notice an increase in the number of days when she experiences some type of mucus. As suckling is reduced, the body will increasingly try to ovulate until it succeeds. During this process the woman will experience a greater number of days of wet, somewhat slippery mucus.
5. Days of bleeding may even occur. Since mucus can be mixed in with the blood, *it is very important to treat the days of bleeding — even slight spotting — as fertile mucus days and to abstain from intercourse.*

The breastfeeding woman who is either not ovulating or ovulating occasionally needs to follow the alternate dry day and mucus patch rules.*

As with women experiencing anovulation for other reasons, observation of the cervix can prove helpful.

Some women who breastfeed and some women approaching menopause experience an extremely dry feeling in the vaginal canal. The loss of the usual moisture in these tissues is due to a lack of the estrogen usually present in large amounts with ovulatory cycles. If the vaginal tissues become dry, intercourse and

*If you are interested in learning about total breastfeeding and how to prolong anovulation, we suggest reading *Natural Breastfeeding and Childspacing* by Sheila Kippley. See the Bibliography for this book and other books on breastfeeding.

urination can be uncomfortable or painful. A woman should talk with her doctor if this change in the vagina takes place.

Moist vaginal tissue helps cervical mucus travel down to the vaginal opening. Dry vaginal tissue does not aid the flow of mucus. A woman in this situation may find it helpful to use internal checking in combination with external checking. For example, the woman approaching menopause who experiences this type of menopausal dryness can benefit from checking for mucus that may be present at the opening of the cervix. If the woman in this situation experiences a dry vaginal sensation and no mucus with external checking, yet with internal checking observes the presence of wet mucus, she should continue to check internally. Her dry vaginal tissue is slowing down the flow of wet mucus; therefore, internal checking may be more effective.

How to Check for Mucus Internally:

1. Insert 2 fingers into the vagina until you feel the cervix.
2. Place one finger on each side of the cervix.
3. Gently press your fingers against the cervix.
4. Move your fingers to the opening of the cervix to collect mucus.
5. Remove your fingers and slowly stretch them apart.
6. Observe the amount, color and quality of the mucus.

A word about basal body temperature for new mothers, women approaching menopause and all other women experiencing anovulation.

We realize that taking the basal body temperature every day may not be convenient. If the temperature cannot be taken every day, we strongly suggest taking it as soon as there is an appearance of wet mucus or a change in the basic infertile pattern. If the thermal shift occurs when there has been a mucus pattern that changes to ovulatory, wet, stretchy mucus, the thermal shift and peak day rules can be applied to determine the beginning of the absolutely infertile phase. However, until a woman has resumed ovulating for 6 cycles in a row, the calculated infertile phase rule cannot be applied.

For example, Carmen has ovulated for the first time after one year of breastfeeding. She is now able to use the thermal shift and peak day rules. Yet until her fertility signs give proof of ovulation for 6 cycles in a row, she would consider herself fertile during any type of bleeding and continue to use the alternate dry day rule and mucus patch rule until the beginning of the absolutely infertile phase.

You will be able to recognize anovulation and prevent pregnancy through careful observation of fertility signs. Missing periods for several months in no way harms the body. However, if a woman has not experienced periods for more than 3 months for reasons other than total breastfeeding, we suggest that she discuss this situation with her doctor.

TO REVIEW:

Basal Body Temperature

- *A woman who ovulates will see her temperature shift from low to high.*
- *A woman who does not ovulate will not see her temperature shift from low to high.*

Cervical Mucus

- *A woman who ovulates will develop very wet, slippery, stretchy mucus as she approaches ovulation.*
- *A woman who does not ovulate will not develop the true wet, stretchy mucus. She can experience a variety of mucus patterns from all dry days to a combination of wet-feeling mucus, sticky mucus and dry days throughout the entire time she does not ovulate.*

Cervical Changes

- *A woman who ovulates will experience a cervix that rises to a high position, becomes soft and opens wide.*
- *A woman who does not ovulate will experience a cervix that either remains low, firm and closed or that rises slightly, becomes slightly soft and slightly open.*

Secondary Fertility Signs

- *A woman who ovulates will notice one sign or more which shows she is ovulating.*
- *A woman who is not ovulating will not experience her usual secondary fertility signs.*

Remember, if you have anovulatory cycles that continue beyond 3 months, it is important to discuss this with your physician. It is also helpful to take all of your fertility awareness charts to the physician as they can help him/her to better understand your particular situation.

Other Special Circumstances

After Childbirth

If you are not breastfeeding, you may begin ovulating within 2 weeks after the delivery. If you want to use your fertility signs to prevent pregnancy, you should begin observing your mucus and temperature as soon after the delivery as possible. It can be difficult for you to observe your fertility signs if you are a new mother, awakening at irregular times to take care of your new baby, etc. However, you should try to begin checking your mucus and cervix when the discharge from childbirth has stopped. This discharge is called lochia. It can be very difficult, if not impossible, to check mucus with this discharge present. Usually, 3 weeks after delivery the lochia has stopped and observation of the mucus and cervix can begin. Also by this time you should begin observing your temperature.

Vaginal Infection

Another common special circumstance is a vaginal infection. One of the symptoms of a vaginal infection is the presence of a discharge from the vagina that looks different from the normal vaginal and cervical secretions. The second symptom can be an odor in the vaginal area that is unlike the usual vaginal scent. A third symptom can be burning and/or itching in the vaginal area. If you experience one or more symptoms, it is important for you to be examined to identify the cause of the infection and receive proper treatment.

During the time of a vaginal infection you will have difficulty observing your mucus changes, particularly if you are using a medication in the form of a vaginal cream or suppository. However, you can still continue to take your basal body temperature. It is not advisable to check your cervix or have intercourse until the vaginal infection has cleared up. If the infection is healed by the time you have accurately applied the thermal shift rule, you can safely resume intercourse.

Premenstrual Tension Syndrome

Premenstrual tension syndrome (PMTS) is the name given to various troubling emotional and/or physical changes experienced by many women, lasting anywhere from 1 to 14 days, usually before menstruation begins. (Some women also seem to experience the changes only during menstruation and for a couple of days after menstruation ends.)

There are perhaps 150 different signals known as premenstrual symptoms that let a woman know she is approaching the time of menstrual bleeding. The most common of these symptoms are: nervous tension; mood swings; irritability; anxiety; headache; craving for sweets; increased appetite; heart pounding; fatigue; dizziness or fainting; depression; forgetfulness; crying; confusion; insomnia, weight gain; swelling of hands, feet and legs; breast tenderness; and abdominal bloating.

The research conducted about PMTS has shown that this problem is probably due to an imbalance in estrogen and progesterone. It seems that some women with PMTS have more than the normal amount of estrogen combined with an amount of progesterone that is less than normal. A rarer form of PMTS is one in which the opposite is true. A woman with this kind of PMTS has too little estrogen and enough or too much progesterone.

Regardless of the amounts of estrogen and progesterone a woman has, an imbalance in these hormones appears to cause the brain and other parts of the body to go haywire. The brain puts out abnormal amounts of special chemicals that affect the way a woman thinks and feels as well as contribute to the body's tendency to "hold water."

We could go on and discuss other research that has recently begun, research related to brain and body chemistry that might end up unraveling all the causes of PMTS. However, it is too early to draw any conclusions. Therefore, we will be more concerned with the important question women are asking, "What can a woman do to help herself?" Another question to address is, "Does PMTS affect the use of NFP and FAM?"

Does PMTS affect the use of NFP and FAM?

Picture the woman who has applied the absolutely infertile phase rules to enable her to know when the egg is dead and gone. She resumes having intercourse or puts her method of birth control away, only to find that the day after ovulation or a few days after ovulation, she begins to experience breast tenderness, bloating, headaches and fatigue. Does she now feel like having intercourse? Probably not! In other words, the woman following NFP or FAM who experiences PMTS may have an absolutely infertile phase partially or totally filled with physical and/or emotional changes that cause her to be turned off to any kind of sexual activity. What then does the absolutely infertile phase have to offer her if she doesn't want to use it?

In addition to how the woman feels, her fertility signs may show the results of PMTS. We have observed slow rising temperature patterns, irregular mucus patterns and temperature which does not stay up for 12 to 16 days in some women with PMTS. Whether the patterns of fertility signs are a bit or severely irregular due to PMTS in every woman that has it, is something no one knows. Therefore, a woman should try to rid herself of this hormonal imbalance so that she can feel better, and if her fertility signs are affected, they will probably be clearer to identify if the problem is corrected.

Treating PMTS

It is quite common for some women to experience physical and emotional changes from caffeine, sugar, alcohol, and salt in their diets. Most women can begin to help themselves by following these nutritional guidelines:

- Limit eating refined sugar to 5 tablespoons a day (if you have to eat any sugar).
- Limit alcohol to 1 ounce a day (if you have to drink an alcoholic beverage).
- Do not drink more than 1 cup of coffee or tea or an 8-ounce can of a soft drink with caffeine a day.
- Limit tobacco use.
- Limit intake of red meat to 3 ounces a day.
- Rely more on fish, poultry, whole grains and legumes as sources of protein and less on red meat and dairy products.
- Eat leafy green vegetables and fresh fruit every day.
- Use 2 tablespoons uncooked safflower oil on salads or vegetables every day.

These guidelines for exercise and relaxation can also help:

- Take a 20-minute walk every day. Walking is a non-stress exercise that can build up strength, be relaxing and get you out in the fresh air on a regular basis.
- If there is considerable stress in your life, deciding on a way to help decrease the stress can help, for example, talking with a counselor or therapist, meditating, listening to music, taking up a hobby, etc. A woman can benefit greatly from learning what helps her to relax and handle stressful situations better.

Many women also often benefit greatly from taking vitamins and minerals. Some research has shown that estrogen and progesterone may not be present in normal amounts because a woman is not taking in enough of all the B vitamins and magnesium.[1] Dr. Gui Abraham, a gynecologist and researcher of premenstrual problems for the past thirteen years, suggests the following well-balanced *total* vitamin and mineral program to help relieve premenstrual symptoms. Women with mild symptoms may need only one-half the amounts of the vitamins and minerals listed here. Women with moderate to severe symptoms would probably benefit by taking the full amounts.[2]

Vitamins

Vitamin A	12,500 IU
Vitamin E (d-alpha tocopherol acid succ.)	100 IU
Vitamin D_3 (cholecalciferol)	100 IU
Folic Acid	200 mcg
Vitamin B_1 (thiamine mononitrate)	25 mg
Vitamin B_2 (riboflavin)	25 mg
Niacinamide	25 mg
Vitamin B_6	300 mg
Vitamin B_{12}	62.5 mcg
Biotin	62.5 mcg
Pantothenic acid	25 mg
Inositol	25 mg
Choline Bitartrate	312.5 mg
Para-amino benzoic acid	25 mg
Bioflavonoids	250 mg
Vitamin C (ascorbic acid)	1500 mg
Rutin	25 mg

IU — International Units
mcg — micrograms
mg — milligrams

All the vitamins except Vitamin A, Vitamin E, and Vitamin D_3 should be taken in sustained release form.

Minerals

Calcium	125 mg
Magnesium	250 mg
Iodine	75 mcg
Iron	15 mg
Copper	0.5 mg
Zinc	25 mg
Manganese	10 mg
Potassium	47.5 mg
Selenium	100 mcg
Chromium	100 mcg

All minerals should be taken in chelated form.

In addition, it is helpful to add digestive enzymes to aid the body in absorbing vitamins and minerals. These enzymes include:

Amylase Activity	15,000 USP units
Protease Activity	15,000 USP units
Lipase Activity	1,200 USP units
Betaine Acid HCL	100 mg

It is felt that the B vitamins and all the other vitamins and minerals work together to help the liver break down estrogen and sugar. When these are broken down and used well by the body, the chances of female hormones, sugar, and brain chemistry imbalance are reduced.

TIPS ON VITAMINS AND MINERALS

- Take them with a meal.
- Take them *every day.*
- Urine will probably be darker yellow in color and have a stronger than usual smell while you are taking them.
- Intestinal gas can occur if a woman is not eating enough whole grains.
- Vitamins and minerals work better if a woman is eating well, exercising regularly, and getting fresh air at least 20 minutes a day, four days a week.

[1] Gui Abraham, M.D., "Premenstrual Tension," *Current Problems in Obstetrics and Gynecology* III August, 1980.

[2] Ibid.

Progesterone therapy is another approach, as well as the use of various drugs, for the treatment of PMTS. Again, research is limited as to whether drugs and hormones really work for every woman with PMTS. If a woman wishes to use progesterone or certain drugs, it is an extremely good idea to combine this drug therapy with a sound nutritional, exercise and vitamin and mineral program.*

Some women have stated that when they have decreased the amount of mucus-producing foods (for example, dairy foods) in their diets, they have noticed a decrease in the amount of cervical mucus produced. Other women who have needed to take prescription antihistamines, drugs that dry up the secretions in the nasal passages, notice a drying up of their mucus.

You can be aware of those factors that might affect your own mucus pattern. If you change your diet or need to take certain drugs and see a change in your mucus pattern, with careful observation you will probably be able to utilize your mucus to avoid pregnancy. If you experience a substantial decrease in mucus or a constant dry feeling, yet you know you are ovulating by seeing a thermal shift, you may need to use internal checking. If you find yourself confused or concerned, talking with your doctor, as well as having a physical examination, will be helpful. It may also be valuable to seek advice from a fertility awareness instructor.

As you can see, just about every woman can observe her fertility signs as a means of pregnancy avoidance. If you experience a special circumstance, be on the lookout for signs of fertility and follow the rules carefully. At first some women find these rules somewhat confusing. But please remember that the language your body speaks is a clear, accurate language. The time and effort you spend will enable you to understand it. We hope you will be encouraged, for the language is worth the learning.

*Remember to see the Bibliography for books that discuss PMTS.

notes:

CHAPTER XI

PUTTING IT ALL TOGETHER
THE FERTILITY AWARENESS METHOD WAY
Rules for Avoiding Pregnancy

Some things catch on because they are fads; other ideas catch on because they are sound, valuable and workable.

Fertility Awareness Method (FAM) is such a concept. Increasingly couples are turning away from the pill and IUD toward barrier and/or spermicidal methods. And some couples are turning away from barrier and/or spermicidal methods toward FAM. The reason for the change to FAM is both reasonable and simple.

It is reasonable because it is based on natural body awareness, and it is simple because the information you need to follow is always with you.

Couples who have been using barrier methods of birth control (condom, diaphragm and cervical cap) and couples who have been using spermicides (jelly, creams, foam and suppositories) *now have an alternative so they don't have to use these methods each time they have intercourse.* FAM is based on the same scientific principles as natural family planning, yet FAM offers an alternative to abstaining from intercourse during the fertile days of the menstrual cycle. This means that *only during fertile days is it necessary to use another method of birth control.* Therefore, the number of days these methods are necessary can be greatly decreased.

Traditionally, men and women have learned that a method of birth control must be used every time they have intercourse. This is not necessary since the number of fertile days during each cycle averages from 5 to 7. A couple having intercourse during this time can use any of the methods mentioned above. In other words, FAM offers another choice in avoiding pregnancy.

Fertility awareness method offers choices and options. The options or variations you choose depend on the barrier and/or spermicidal method of birth control you wish to use and on the fertility signs you wish to observe.

The way in which FAM is used also depends upon how you feel about using the other methods of birth control. For example, Judy has been using the diaphragm for 2 years. Although she is basically satisfied with it, she and her partner have been talking about changing their method of birth control to one that does not interrupt their lovemaking. They feel that at times the diaphragm does not allow them the freedom they would like to have with intercourse. This couple decided to give FAM a chance. Judy learned how to determine her fertile and infertile phases. Once she learned this, she and her partner no longer needed to use the diaphragm each time they had intercourse. Now that they need to use the diaphragm less often, they no longer feel the need to change their method of birth control.

We have already discussed the factors which prevent you from accurately observing your cervical mucus. One of these factors is spermicidal preparations. These chemicals, when inserted into the vagina with or without the diaphragm, condom or cervical cap, kill the sperm. They also cover up cervical mucus. Therefore, if you choose to use a spermicide, you will be unable to observe your mucus changes during the days when the spermicide is present in your vagina. However, the fertility sign which can be observed is your basal body temperature.

How can you minimize the use of birth control methods after ovulation? The basal body temperature can be used with or without cervical changes. Observation of the basal body temperature used with the application of the thermal shift rule can provide you with a way to identify the absolutely infertile Phase III. Once this phase begins, a method of birth control is no longer necessary until the beginning of the next menstrual cycle.

For example, a woman can use contraceptive foam until she can apply the thermal shift rule. Once the absolutely infertile phase begins, she no longer needs to use the contraceptive foam for the remainder of that menstrual cycle. Knowing when the absolutely infertile phase begins eliminates the need for birth control for about 10 days of the menstrual cycle.

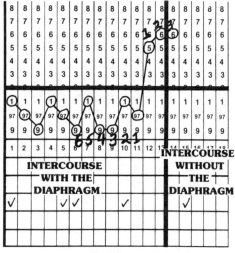

Figure 47—Diaphragm use and the Thermal Shift Rule

In Figure 47 — Carmen did not want to use the calculated infertile phase rule. Instead she used her diaphragm whenever she had intercourse until she determined she was no longer fertile. Because she was using the diaphragm, she chose to observe only her basal body temperature. By applying the thermal shift rule, her absolutely infertile phase began on the evening of cycle day 14. From that evening through the remainder of that menstrual cycle, she could have intercourse safely without the need for her diaphragm.

Another example of how FAM can be applied is the use of the non-lubricated condom in combination with cervical mucus and basal body temperature observations. Because the condom prevents semen from entering the vagina, the cervical mucus is not affected. Use of the condom allows accurate observation of mucus changes and successful application of the peak day rule. For instance, a couple may use the non-lubricated condom until the thermal shift and peak day rules are applied to determine the beginning of the absolutely infertile phase. Once this phase begins, the condom is not needed for the remainder of that menstrual cycle.

How can you minimize the use of birth control methods before ovulation? The calculated infertile Phase I rule can be used just as it is in natural family planning to provide you with days for intercourse before ovulation that are 95 to 99% safe from pregnancy.

Here are some typical cases:

If your last 6 menstrual cycles were 30, 31, 30, 29, 30 and 29 days long, by subtracting 21 from the shortest of the 6 cycles you have a calculated infertile Phase I of 8 days (29 - 21 = 8). The first 8 days of your menstrual cycle can be used to have intercourse without another method of birth control. When the fertile Phase II begins and if you choose to have intercourse, you can utilize another method of birth control until you can successfully apply the thermal shift rule (and if possible apply the peak day rule). Once the absolutely infertile Phase III begins, you no longer need to use your other method of birth control for the remainder of the menstrual cycle.

To reduce the pregnancy rate during the calculated infertile Phase I, the true menses rule and the alternate dry day rule can be used, as explained in Chapter 9. The alternate dry day rule can only be applied if you

are able to check for the presence or absence of mucus. The non-lubricated condom is the only method that enables you to watch for the presence of early warning mucus which could indicate an early ovulation.

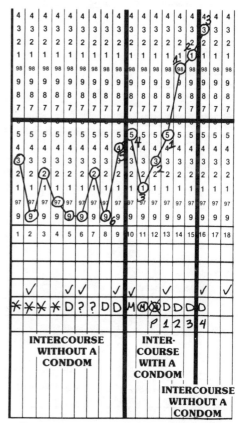

Figure 48—Condom use, the Calculated Infertile Phase, and Thermal Shift

In Figure 48 — Chris has a calculated infertile phase of 9 days. During that time she and Nicki had intercourse without using a method of contraception. Since they wished to have intercourse after the start of the fertile phase on day 10, they used a non-lubricated condom. Use of the condom enabled them to observe the cervical mucus changes. They continued to use a condom until they could apply the peak day and thermal shift rules. Once the absolutely infertile phase began on the evening of cycle day 16, they continued having intercourse, but without the need for a condom the remainder of that menstrual cycle.

As you can see, there are a variety of ways in which fertility signs, rules and other methods of birth control can be combined to avoid pregnancy.

Contraceptive methods can be used during the fertile phase only or during the calculated infertile and fertile phases. It all depends on how great the desire is to avoid pregnancy and to decrease the use of another method of birth control.

As discussed in Chapter 2, it is generally believed that the pregnancy rates with FAM should not be any higher than the rates are when using the barrier and/or spermicidal methods alone, providing the rules are followed carefully.

Your willingness to observe your fertility signs and use the birth control methods conscientiously are the key to FAM. Because intercourse is taking place during the fertile phase — the phase with the highest risk of pregnancy — the careful and consistent use of the methods is of utmost importance if pregnancy is to be avoided.

notes:

CHAPTER XII

ACHIEVING A PREGNANCY AND FACTS ABOUT INFERTILITY

Many have mistakenly assumed a woman could become pregnant at any time during her menstrual cycle. However, as you have learned from previous chapters, a woman has only a few fertile days when pregnancy is possible.

Therefore, *if a couple want to have a baby, they must have intercourse during the fertile phase of the menstrual cycle.*

Instructions for Planning a Pregnancy

Ideally you should take the time to observe your fertility signs (at least cervical mucus and basal body temperature) for a month or more before you want to achieve a pregnancy. By doing this you will become familiar with your changing mucus and temperature patterns. Knowing these patterns can enable you to become familiar with your fertile days and to be able to determine them during future menstrual cycles. If you learn about your fertility patterns before pregnancy, you can develop the understanding necessary to use your fertility signs to avoid pregnancy after the baby is born.

Once you've observed your fertility signs for at least one menstrual cycle, *you should begin having intercourse on the first day of a wet vaginal sensation and wet mucus. Intercourse should continue every other day during the wet sensations and mucus.* Abstaining from intercourse for 48 hours maximizes the number of sperm in the man's semen.

Having intercourse close to the time of the rise in your basal body temperature gives you the greatest possibility of pregnancy. However, since you cannot predict the exact day that your temperature will rise, *the wet cervical mucus is the best indicator of the beginning of the fertile time.* If you are observing your cervical changes, a high, soft and open cervix is another indication of the fertile days.

Once your temperature shifts, you should continue taking it for the remainder of the cycle. If your basal body temperature remains high longer than 20 days and you don't experience your usual menstrual bleeding, it usually means that you are pregnant. If you have any indications of pregnancy, it is important that you have a pregnancy test and be examined so that the pregnancy can be confirmed and the date the baby will be born can be determined. Another reason for this examination is the need to begin early obstetrical care for the health of the mother and baby.

TO REVIEW:

1. *Observe your fertility signs for one cycle or more. If you want to learn about the mucus pattern, abstinence from intercourse or use of a non-lubricated condom during these cycles will enable accurate observation of the mucus changes.*
2. *Once you've decided to become pregnant, intercourse should take place once the wet, fertile mucus begins.*
3. *Having intercourse every other day maximizes the number of sperm in the semen.*
4. *Continue taking your basal body temperature after the rise. A temperature which remains elevated beyond the usual cycle length is an excellent sign that pregnancy has been achieved.*

Intercourse must occur during wet mucus days to achieve pregnancy, but it doesn't mean intercourse shouldn't take place during other days in the cycle. Some couples "trying to become pregnant" change their usual sexual lifestyle in a way that isn't pleasing to them. Instead of enjoying each other sexually whenever they desire, they abstain from intercourse and from other ways of being affectionate during non-fertile times of the menstrual cycle.

There is no reason why intercourse can't take place at any time early in the menstrual cycle. However, since you want to be able to detect the first day of wet mucus and a wet vaginal sensation, having intercourse every other day will enable you to observe the wet mucus. Abstinence for one day after intercourse provides the time needed for semen to leave the vaginal area. This will enable a woman to accurately determine the beginning of the wet mucus production.

In addition to learning fertility signs and proper timing for intercourse, the couple desiring a pregnancy should consider a few other issues.

First, it is important to have a complete medical checkup before becoming pregnant. This examination gives you and your doctor an opportunity to discuss any medical problems that might exist. For example, if you are taking medications, it is important to know if they will be harmful if taken during pregnancy. An examination will also provide the opportunity, if necessary, for certain tests, such as Rubella (German measles), Sickle Cell Anemia and Tay-Sachs Disease, to be performed.

Another issue is selection of the child's sex through special methods of timing intercourse. Several sources have stated that pregnancy occurring as a result of intercourse a few days before the thermal shift (in other words, when wet mucus first appears) increases the possibility of the baby being a girl. Intercourse occurring near the day of the thermal shift and/or day of the most abundant wet, slippery mucus increases the possibility of a boy.

Although studies have been conducted and books have been written on this subject, planning the child's sex presently seems to be successful for only a small percentage of those couples who have tried to do so.*

Infertility

Approximately 15% of all couples have some difficulty achieving a pregnancy. Unfortunately, many of them don't know when to seek medical attention, and they are unaware of the facts about infertility tests and treatments. Other couples delay seeking medical attention because of fear. They are fearful of having a problem that cannot be corrected. Some are not aware that there are successful treatments for many causes of infertility.

On the average, it takes a couple 3 to 4 months to achieve a pregnancy. About 85% of couples attempting to achieve a pregnancy will succeed after one year of "trying." There are many reasons why the other 15% do not succeed. Some causes are due to problems with the man. Others are due to problems with the woman. Occasionally, both the man and the woman will have problems. If a couple has not achieved a pregnancy after having intercourse on the fertile days for 6 to 9 menstrual cycles, they should seek help from a physician who treats fertility problems.

*See the Bibliography for books about selecting the sex of a baby.

Infertility and the Man

The most common problems are related either to a low number of sperm in the semen or poor activity (movement) of the sperm. The causes of these problems include:

- infection
- exposure to chemicals
- medical illnesses
- prescription and non-prescription drugs
- dilated veins in the scrotum (varicocele)

Other causes of infertility are abnormalities of the testes and the passageways necessary for the normal travel of sperm and seminal fluid. These abnormalities can be due to improperly developed parts of the reproductive system, infection or operations in or near the genital area.

The first test used to check the number and quality of sperm is called *semen analysis*. If the test is not normal, additional special tests and procedures are performed to identify the cause and possible treatment of the problem. If the semen analysis is normal, then infertility testing of the woman is begun.

Infertility and the Woman

Anovulation — no ovulation or infrequent ovulation — is a common cause of infertility in women that is often successfully treated by the use of medication. This problem is due to one or both of the following causes:

- disturbances in the usual ways the hormones are supposed to work
- physical and emotional stress (discussed in Chapter 10)

Another cause of infertility is cervical problems. Cervical infections or surgery performed on the cervix can lead to:

- inadequate production of cervical mucus
- production of cervical mucus that may not be of the quality necessary to allow sperm to live and pass through it to reach the egg

Cervical mucus can also contain substances that inactivate the sperm, in the manner the body produces antibodies that inactivate bacteria and viruses when it is "fighting off" an infection or illness. Common treatments for these problems include:

- antibiotics to clear up infections
- estrogen treatment to increase the amount and improve the quality of the mucus

Problems of the uterus and fallopian tubes are also causes for infertility. An infection occurring in and around the internal reproductive organs (pelvic infection) can cause scarring of the fallopian tubes. This scarring may prevent the sperm from reaching the egg or the egg from entering the tube. Sometimes this can be corrected by tubal surgery.

Endometriosis (endo-me-tree-o-sis) is a cause of infertility that occurs more often in older women who have delayed having children. It is believed the endometriosis develops when the tissue which normally lines the inside of the uterus flows up through the fallopian tubes into the area of the ovaries. The presence of this tissue can cause scarring that may prevent the sperm from reaching the egg or the egg from entering the tube. Endometriosis can be treated by surgery to remove the tissue and scarring. Hormone therapy is another treatment used to reduce growth of the endometrial tissue.

Other Causes of Infertility

Approximately 5% of all couples who have an infertility evaluation will show no identifiable cause for their infertility. Some of these couples will achieve a pregnancy at some time without treatment of any kind. For others who have particularly stressful life situations, pregnancy may occur after they have dealt successfully with their stress. Some are able to do this by themselves, while others may need to seek the assistance of a professional skilled in helping people emotionally — a psychologist, counselor or psychiatrist.

Improper Timing of Intercourse

It may take a prolonged period of time for a couple to achieve a pregnancy simply because they are unaware of the fertile phase of the menstrual cycle. Observing fertility signs can often enable a couple to achieve a pregnancy sooner because they are aware of the woman's fertile time.

Feelings and Infertility

Infertility is usually an extremely difficult life situation for a couple. Since many women and men have a strong desire for a child, the couple unable to have a child of their own may experience feelings of anger and frustration, as well as guilt, depression and sadness. These feelings can be devastating to the couple and their relationship. Because of this, it can be helpful to talk with someone who can provide support and understanding. An infertility organization, therapist, counselor or religious leader can provide this support and be of benefit to couples working through this very difficult time.

We have chosen not to discuss all of the many tests, causes and treatments of fertility problems. This is not because we don't feel it is important. Our reason is quite the opposite. A thorough discussion of infertility deserves its

own book.   An example of such a book is
Infertility Guide for the Childless Couple by
Barbara Eck Menning.*

*See the Bibliography for this book and others about infertility.

notes:

CHAPTER XIII

THE ADVANTAGES AND DISADVANTAGES OF NATURAL FAMILY PLANNING AND FERTILITY AWARENESS METHODS

The majority of this book has been about facts. Facts about the reproductive organs, the menstrual cycle, fertility signs and rules. We hope what you have learned has been valuable for you and that you will be able to use all of these facts in many rewarding ways.

Knowing these facts can help you discover how you feel about yourself, your sexuality and pregnancy. This is what this chapter is about . . . feelings . . . feelings about fertility and sexuality and what these feelings mean to you. This is of great importance because your feelings will determine what the possible advantages and disadvantages of natural family planning will be for you.

Should You Use Natural Family Planning?

A conscious decision to use NFP, or any method of birth control for that matter, is one that only you can make. Taking time to personally examine the advantages and disadvantages of NFP will help you to answer the very important question of whether or not you should use it as your method of birth control.

Advantages. . .

- NFP is not physically harmful.
- It promotes an understanding of the fertility cycle.
- It can be used by the woman who has truly irregular menstrual cycles, is breast-feeding or premenopausal.
- NFP is as effective in avoiding pregnancy, if used properly, as most of the other birth control methods.
- It requires the man's cooperation and mutual sharing of responsibility for fertility control. NFP can promote a greater understanding of one another's sexual and emotional needs, and it can enhance a couple's love and respect for each other.
- In addition, it is an inexpensive means of birth control.

Disadvantages. . .

- NFP requires more time to learn and use than other birth control methods.
- It requires the cooperation of the man.
- It may require a change in sexual life-style since abstinence during the fertile days is necessary.
- Because it requires more cooperation from the man, NFP is not used properly as often as the pill and IUD. Therefore, in actual use it is not as effective as the pill and IUD.

What may be experienced as an advantage for some may seem to be a disadvantage for others. For example, if the man finds it difficult to abstain during the fertile days and is not supportive of fertility sign observation and charting, then the relationship may be disrupted. Or if the man wants to use NFP and the woman finds it difficult to abstain during the fertile days, likewise the relationship may be disrupted. However, when there is mutual commitment to abstinence, the relationship is often enhanced.

If you are considering NFP as a method of avoiding pregnancy, an important question to ask yourself is: Can you reach a mutual agreement with your partner to abstain from intercourse periodically and feel good about this way of avoiding pregnancy?

For many this may be a difficult question to answer. It can be helpful when trying, to consider if in your relationship you are able to talk together openly and honestly about how to avoid pregnancy.

If your relationship is one in which effective and satisfying communication about sexuality and fertility control cannot occur, it does not mean it will always be that way. In a relationship a man and woman learn, grow and change. And fortunately, there are ways to help the growing process so people can experience and enjoy the kinds of relationships they want.

With so many social changes rapidly taking place in our society, there is a great opportunity for women and men to learn about themselves and their sexuality. This new awareness can enable them to make more responsible decisions than ever before.

What Does Sexuality Mean?

For some, sexuality means "intercourse only" — an activity for the main purpose of baby-making. For others, it means a variety of ways of physical pleasuring. And for others, it has a different meaning, including more than sexual activity. This broader definition includes all of the physical and emotional aspects of being a man or a woman — the way a person walks, talks, dresses, makes love, the household duties a person chooses to do, as well as the type of job someone has.

Keeping this broader definition in mind, let's take a look at how we learn about sexuality. Learning about sexuality begins at birth and continues throughout our lifetimes. This learning is influenced by everything and everyone around us. Unfortunately, much of the learning involves information that is usually incorrect or incomplete, and it often gives us messages that our genitals are "dirty" and that sex is something to be hidden. As children we tried to learn what sex was all about. Often this "learning" was done in "secret," behind the garage, in the attic or in the basement. Then as puberty approached, our bodies began to change. These changes, such as menstruation, breast development, sexual feelings, wet dreams, pubic hair and pimples, often created uncomfortable and frightening feelings.

Somehow, as if by magic, in adolescence we were expected to have healthy, mature attitudes about our bodies, sexuality and ourselves. Finally, as adults, we are expected to be knowledgeable, sensitive and comfortable about our sexuality and to take responsibility for our sexuality and fertility. This is not easy when so many of us received a great deal of misinformation and many negative messages about our sexuality.

Misinformation and negative messages are major reasons why people either do not use birth control, or use it improperly. For example, a woman and man who are uncomfortable about their own sexuality often do not take responsibility for avoiding pregnancy, even though they are having intercourse. When an accidental pregnancy occurs, many women say, "I didn't know it (intercourse) was going to happen" or "I didn't think I could get pregnant." The man often says, "It was her fault. She should have done something to prevent the pregnancy."

Misinformation and negative messages not only contribute to unplanned pregnancies, but also can lead to sexual concerns and difficulties. These concerns include many types of dissatisfaction during lovemaking, from the woman who wants an orgasm yet doesn't achieve one, to the man who is unable to have or keep an erection.

Other common reasons for sexual dissatisfaction are disagreement about the times to make love, how long it should last and the type of sexual activity that occurs. For example, a woman may prefer sex in the morning, while her partner may prefer sex in the evening.

It is estimated that 9 out of 10 couples experience dissatisfaction at some time during their relationship because of a lack of accurate information about sex and the failure of the woman and man to communicate sexual feelings.

When uncertain of the facts about sex, people are often afraid to discuss it. Asking questions about sex and talking with a partner, doctor, friend or counselor can be difficult. A person may fear sounding foolish or abnormal in some way. To some, talking with a partner means acknowledging unhappiness with their lovemaking. Because of this, a person may be afraid that his or her partner will feel hurt or become angry.

What we are saying is that there are very real reasons why people aren't open with their feelings. Yet, this doesn't mean they shouldn't try. Once women and men begin to talk about their feelings, they are often amazed to find that their partners have many of the same questions and fears. By sharing these thoughts, they become closer, which helps to enhance not only their sexual lives, but other aspects of their relationship as well.

Many couples have also found that by talking, planning and agreeing on how they want their sexual life to be, they set aside time for giving each other attention and pleasure.

Do You Want a Pregnancy?

This is one of the major questions related to fertility and sexuality that doesn't get asked or decided on as frequently as it should be. The answer to this question is determined by many factors since people decide to have children for different reasons.

There are many reasons why people want children. Some of the reasons can be disruptive to the relationship, while others lead to the development of a loving and happy family.

- "To share our love with another human being."
- "We have so much to give."
- "A woman isn't a woman until she has a child."
- "A man isn't a man until he has a child."
- "To have someone to love."

- "To carry on the family name."
- "To give parents grandchildren."
- "It's normal and expected."

Some men and women see a child as a solution to a problem in their lives.

- "Having a baby will keep us together."
- "Having a baby will keep my wife in her place."
- "Having a baby will make my husband happy, even if I don't want a child right now."
- "Nothing seems to help these lonely feelings I have."
- "I'm nothing unless I am a mother/father."

Having a child can be one of the most wonderful and gratifying experiences in life. Yet, the decision to have a child should not be one that is taken lightly. It requires a great deal of thought, for it is about whether or not a couple have reached a time in their lives when they can care for and love each other, as well as another human being.

Just as there are many reasons why people choose to have a child, there are also many reasons why couples choose to avoid having a child, at least for a period of time.

- "I can't provide for another person at this time in my life."
- "I feel emotionally fulfilled with the child/ children I have."
- "Having a child right now would take time away from developing our relationship."

The decision to avoid or achieve a pregnancy may be difficult to make. Yet, it must be made if any method of birth control is to be used effectively.

It is known that during certain situations, when a couple have not firmly decided upon a birth control method, unplanned pregnancies frequently occur. These include a holiday, vacation, a romantic evening and an occasion where drugs or alcohol are used. When people are relaxed and not feeling the stress in their lives, life's responsibilities and demands do not seem as great, and the desire for sexual pleasure can be increased. Because of these feelings, women often become pregnant, since at that time having a baby seems like the right thing to do. Unfortunately, after the vacation is over or the effects of the alcohol have worn off, the stresses of real life return and the pregnancy is often viewed as a tragedy.

Not only do unplanned pregnancies frequently occur during these situations but often result when a woman or man is experiencing major life changes. Such changes include a separation from a marriage or relationship, graduation from high school or college, dissatisfaction with a job or career, feelings of loneliness or other times of unhappiness. Men and women have been known to think that having a child will be the answer to these problems.

We've discussed some of the facts about sexuality, reasons people have for avoiding and achieving pregnancy, as well as many of the situations in life which commonly lead to pregnancy.

We feel (and perhaps you will agree) that fertility and sexuality play a major role in determining who we are and what we do. And like all good things, sometimes there are problems. The reassuring point is that working out the problems can be a rewarding and positive experience.

How Does Natural Family Planning Fit Into All of This?

Many couples who have made the choice to abstain from intercourse during the fertile days have said the sharing in this method has been an enriching experience for their relationship. Many women not involved in a sexual relationship with one particular person have commented that using fertility signs to avoid pregnancy has given them a sense of control of their reproduction. They have also found that when a partner has learned about how they avoid pregnancy, the man is often fascinated by it, desires to learn more and is supportive of the method.

By discussing their feelings, some men and women found that abstinence from intercourse and all sexual activity during their fertile time worked perfectly for them. Others discovered that they chose to enjoy their partners sexually in ways other than intercourse.

Expressing one's sexuality without having intercourse brings other issues to mind about the use of NFP. Abstinence, in its true definition, means to not have intercourse. For some, it also means to not experience other forms of sexual pleasuring, such as oral sex and other forms of sensual touching. For others, it means that fertile days can be sexually enjoyable times without experiencing intercourse. It becomes a time for touching, massaging, caressing and enjoying any type of physical contact that a man and woman feel comfortable with. Others who found sexual contact — without intercourse — during fertile times difficult, frustrating, or against their beliefs, found they were able to share love, affection and enjoyable times without sexual activity.

In fact, it is sad to say, but great to know

that couples often experience a rebirth in their relationship when they can't have intercourse whenever they desire to. By "sad to say" we mean that it is not unusual for a couple to fall into a routine in which they forget to compliment each other, do things for one another and, in general, enjoy each other without sex. Women and men have commented that becoming aware of fertility and sharing the responsibility of birth control in their sexual relationship has given them a new view of their relationship and reasons for being together. A new awakening, so to speak. For many, this new and greater understanding has enhanced their love for each other.

A Word About Fertility Awareness Method. . .

The use of FAM involves all that we've discussed, plus a bit more. Many couples feel that abstinence seems "unnatural" to them and isn't compatible with their lives. Others feel that if a fertile time coincides with a vacation, holiday, birthday or just a day when the woman or man feels sexual, they want to be able to have intercourse, yet not want a pregnancy to result. Many are comfortable with the use of the diaphragm, condom or spermicide and also feel that they benefit from not feeling "tied down" to these methods each time they have intercourse. FAM offers the freedom they want to have.

It is impossible in one chapter to provide all of the available information about sexuality, communication and relationships. However, we wanted to give you some "food for thought" and encouragement so that, if you haven't already, you will begin to do what is important for you — to feel that you are in control of your reproductive and sexual lives in ways that are best for you. We hope you will gain this control. We are discovering more and more that regardless of age, types of relationships or how men and women choose to use fertility awareness information, it has enabled them to learn about themselves and each other.

Through this learning process, they are sharing feelings and mutual responsibility for enjoying their sexuality. They've learned to feel comfortable about the role fertility plays in their lives. We hope you will, too.

notes:

_____

_____

_____

_____

_____

_____

_____

_____

_____

_____

_____

_____

_____

_____

_____

_____

_____

_____

_____

_____

_____

_____

_____

_____

_____

_____

_____

_____

_____

_____

_____

_____

_____

THE CONTRACT

The thought of a birth control contract may sound cold and impersonal, or perhaps somewhat strange to you. Or it may be an exciting concept.

We've chosen to include it because some women and men have found that it helped them to talk with one another in order to make decisions concerning their sexual lives and feelings about pregnancy and birth control.

The nice part of the contract is that it is negotiable. This means that at any time the couple can change it! Let's say one of the partners in a relationship is feeling as though she/he wants to have a child, when 6 months ago that person felt quite the opposite.

The contract can be "pulled out" and discussed, or perhaps changed. A contract can be a helpful way to regularly assess one's personal needs.

Here are examples of two such contracts for use in natural family planning. If they don't quite suit your needs, you may want to write one of your own.

SAMPLE CONTRACT
(For the woman)

I understand that if this method is to work, I must use it carefully and correctly.

Because I know that there are many reasons for taking chances and allowing pregnancy to happen, I will always explore, try to understand and, if I choose, communicate my feelings about what a pregnancy means to me.

I understand that to avoid pregnancy means:
No genital to genital contact (the penis cannot touch the vagina), and
No intercourse during the fertile time.

Because I respect myself and am aware of my responsibility to myself, I agree to abide by this contract.

Should problems arise with the use of the method, or should I change my mind about avoiding pregnancy, I will decide how to best meet my needs and change the contract accordingly.

by:_____   _____
   Signature   Date

SAMPLE CONTRACT
(For the couple)

We understand that if this method is to work, we must use it carefully and correctly.

Because we know that there are many reasons for taking chances and allowing a pregnancy to happen, we will always explore, try to understand and communicate our feelings about what a pregnancy means to us.

We understand that to avoid a pregnancy means:
No genital to genital contact (the penis cannot touch the vagina), and
No intercourse during the fertile time.

Should problems arise with the use of the method, or should one of us change his/her mind about avoiding pregnancy, we will discuss this with each other and mutually agree upon how the contract should be changed.

Attest:

by:_____   _____
   Signature   Date

by:_____   _____
   Signature   Date

FERTILITY AWARENESS

Usual
Time of
Day
_____

Month _____ Year _____ Cycle Number _____ Cycle Variation _____

Basal Body Temperature

99.0 —	99	9	8	7	6	5	4	3	2	1
98.0 —	98	9	8	7	6	5	4	3	2	1
97.0 —	97	9

(Temperature grid with values 99, 9, 8, 7, 6, 5, 4, 3, 2, 1, 98, 9, 8, 7, 6, 5, 4, 3, 2, 1, 97, 9 repeated across columns for cycle days 1–40)

Cycle Day	1	2	3	4	5	6	7	8	9	10	11	12	13	14	15	16	17	18	19	20	21	22	23	24	25	26	27	28	29	30	31	32	33	34	35	36	37	38	39	40
Date																																								
Day																																								
Intercourse																																								
Mucus																																								
Cervix																																								

Notes:
Mucus
Description:

Sensation

Disturbances,
Schedule
Changes, etc.

MUCUS SYMBOLS:

✳ Menses

D Dry
No Mucus
(and dry vaginal
sensation)

M Non-wet Quality
Mucus
(and dry vaginal
sensation)

(Ⓜ) Wet Quality
Mucus
(and wet vaginal
sensation)

(Ⓧ) Last day of
Wet Quality Mucus
(and wet vaginal
sensation)

CERVIX SYMBOLS: ● ● ○ ○ ○ ● ●

FERTILITY AWARENESS

Usual Time of Day

Month _____   Year _____   Cycle Number _____   Cycle Variation _____

Basal Body Temperature

99.0 —

98.0 —

97.0 —

Cycle Day	1	2	3	4	5	6	7	8	9	10	11	12	13	14	15	16	17	18	19	20	21	22	23	24	25	26	27	28	29	30	31	32	33	34	35	36	37	38	39	40
Date																																								
Day																																								
Intercourse																																								
Mucus																																								
Cervix																																								

Notes:
Mucus Description:

Sensation

Disturbances, Schedule Changes, etc.

MUCUS SYMBOLS:

✳ Menses

D Dry No Mucus (and dry vaginal sensation)

M Non-wet Quality Mucus (and dry vaginal sensation)

Ⓜ Wet Quality Mucus (and wet vaginal sensation)

Ⓜ Last day of Wet Quality Mucus (and wet vaginal sensation)

CERVIX SYMBOLS: ● ● ○ ○ ○ ● ●

FERTILITY AWARENESS

Usual Time of Day

Month _____ Year _____ Cycle Number _____ Cycle Variation _____

Basal Body Temperature

99.0	(temperature grid: 99.0, 98.0, 97.0 scale with rows 99, 9, 8, 7, 6, 5, 4, 3, 2, 1 repeating across 40 day columns)

Cycle Day	1	2	3	4	5	6	7	8	9	10	11	12	13	14	15	16	17	18	19	20	21	22	23	24	25	26	27	28	29	30	31	32	33	34	35	36	37	38	39	40
Date																																								
Day																																								
Intercourse																																								
Mucus																																								
Cervix																																								

Notes:
Mucus Description:

Sensation

Disturbances, Schedule Changes, etc.

MUCUS SYMBOLS:

✳ Menses

D — Dry / No Mucus (and dry vaginal sensation)

M — Non-wet Quality Mucus (and dry vaginal sensation)

Ⓜ — Wet Quality Mucus (and wet vaginal sensation)

Ⓜ̸ — Last day of Wet Quality Mucus (and wet vaginal sensation)

CERVIX SYMBOLS: ●● ○ ○ ○ ● ●

FERTILITY AWARENESS

Usual Time of Day ____

Month _____   Year _____   Cycle Number _____   Cycle Variation _____

Basal Body Temperature

Scale	Values across 40 days
	1 (all columns)
99.0	99 9 8 7 6 5 4 3 2 1
98.0	98 9 8 7 6 5 4 3 2 1
97.0	97 9

Cycle Day: 1 2 3 4 5 6 7 8 9 10 11 12 13 14 15 16 17 18 19 20 21 22 23 24 25 26 27 28 29 30 31 32 33 34 35 36 37 38 39 40

Date

Day

Intercourse

Mucus

Cervix

Notes:
  Mucus Description:

  Sensation

Disturbances, Schedule Changes, etc.

MUCUS SYMBOLS:

☀	D	M	Ⓜ	Ⓜ (crossed)
Menses	Dry No Mucus (and dry vaginal sensation)	Non-wet Quality Mucus (and dry vaginal sensation)	Wet Quality Mucus (and wet vaginal sensation)	Last day of Wet Quality Mucus (and wet vaginal sensation)

CERVIX SYMBOLS:

FERTILITY AWARENESS

Usual
Time of
Day

Month _____   Year _____   Cycle Number _____   Cycle Variation _____

Basal Body Temperature

| | 99.0 | | | | | | | | | | | | | | | | | | | | | | | | | | | | | | | | | | | | | | | |

(temperature grid ranging from 99.0 down through 98.0 and 97.0, with rows numbered 1, 99, 9, 8, 7, 6, 5, 4, 3, 2, 1, 98, 9, 8, 7, 6, 5, 4, 3, 2, 1, 97, 9)

Cycle Day	1	2	3	4	5	6	7	8	9	10	11	12	13	14	15	16	17	18	19	20	21	22	23	24	25	26	27	28	29	30	31	32	33	34	35	36	37	38	39	40

Date

Day

Intercourse

Mucus

Cervix

Notes:
Mucus
Description:

Sensation

Disturbances,
Schedule
Changes, etc.

MUCUS SYMBOLS:

✳	D	M	Ⓜ	Ⓧ
Menses	Dry No Mucus (and dry vaginal sensation)	Non-wet Quality Mucus (and dry vaginal sensation)	Wet Quality Mucus (and wet vaginal sensation)	Last day of Wet Quality Mucus (and wet vaginal sensation)

CERVIX SYMBOLS: ● ● ○ O O ○ ● ●

FERTILITY AWARENESS

Usual Time of Day
____

Month _____ Year _____ Cycle Number _____ Cycle Variation _____

Basal Body Temperature

99.0 —

98.0 —

97.0 —

Cycle Day	1	2	3	4	5	6	7	8	9	10	11	12	13	14	15	16	17	18	19	20	21	22	23	24	25	26	27	28	29	30	31	32	33	34	35	36	37	38	39	40
Date																																								
Day																																								
Intercourse																																								
Mucus																																								
Cervix																																								

Notes:
  Mucus Description:

  Sensation

Disturbances, Schedule Changes, etc.

MUCUS SYMBOLS:

✳ Menses

D Dry No Mucus (and dry vaginal sensation)

M Non-wet Quality Mucus (and dry vaginal sensation)

Ⓜ Wet Quality Mucus (and wet vaginal sensation)

Ⓜ̶ Last day of Wet Quality Mucus (and wet vaginal sensation)

CERVIX SYMBOLS: ● ● ∘ ○ ○ ∘ ● ●

FERTILITY AWARENESS

Usual Time of Day ____

Month _____   Year _____   Cycle Number _____   Cycle Variation _____

Basal Body Temperature

Temp																																								
99.0	99 99 99 99 99 99 99 99 99 99 99 99 99 99 99 09 99 99 99 99 99 99 99 99 99 99 99 99 99 99 99 99 99 99 99 99 99 99 99 99
	9 8 7 6 5 4 3 2 1 (rows)
98.0	98 ... 9 8 7 6 5 4 3 2 1 (rows)
97.0	97 ... 9 (rows)

Cycle Day: 1 2 3 4 5 6 7 8 9 10 11 12 13 14 15 16 17 18 19 20 21 22 23 24 25 26 27 28 29 30 31 32 33 34 35 36 37 38 39 40

Date

Day

Intercourse

Mucus

Cervix

Notes:
Mucus Description:

Sensation

Disturbances, Schedule Changes, etc.

MUCUS SYMBOLS:

※ Menses

D Dry No Mucus (and dry vaginal sensation)

M Non-wet Quality Mucus (and dry vaginal sensation)

Ⓜ Wet Quality Mucus (and wet vaginal sensation)

Ⓜ̶ Last day of Wet Quality Mucus (and wet vaginal sensation)

CERVIX SYMBOLS: ● ● ○ ○ ○ ● ● ●

FERTILITY AWARENESS

Month _____   Year _____   Cycle Number _____   Cycle Variation _____

Basal Body Temperature

99.0

98.0

97.0

Cycle Day | 1 | 2 | 3 | 4 | 5 | 6 | 7 | 8 | 9 | 10 | 11 | 12 | 13 | 14 | 15 | 16 | 17 | 18 | 19 | 20 | 21 | 22 | 23 | 24 | 25 | 26 | 27 | 28 | 29 | 30 | 31 | 32 | 33 | 34 | 35 | 36 | 37 | 38 | 39 | 40

Date

Day

Intercourse

Mucus

Cervix

Notes:
Mucus
Description:

Sensation

Disturbances,
Schedule
Changes, etc.

MUCUS SYMBOLS:

✳	D	M	Ⓜ	ⓧ
Menses	Dry No Mucus (and dry vaginal sensation)	Non-wet Quality Mucus (and dry vaginal sensation)	Wet Quality Mucus (and wet vaginal sensation)	Last day of Wet Quality Mucus (and wet vaginal sensation)

CERVIX SYMBOLS: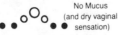

FERTILITY AWARENESS

Usual
Time of
Day

Month _____ Year _____ Cycle Number _____ Cycle Variation _____

Basal Body Temperature

99.0 —

98.0 —

97.0 —

Cycle Day	1	2	3	4	5	6	7	8	9	10	11	12	13	14	15	16	17	18	19	20	21	22	23	24	25	26	27	28	29	30	31	32	33	34	35	36	37	38	39	40

Date

Day

Intercourse

Mucus

Cervix

Notes:
   Mucus
   Description:

   Sensation

Disturbances,
Schedule
Changes, etc.

MUCUS SYMBOLS:

✳	D	M	Ⓜ	Ⓧ
Menses	Dry No Mucus (and dry vaginal sensation)	Non-wet Quality Mucus (and dry vaginal sensation)	Wet Quality Mucus (and wet vaginal sensation)	Last day of Wet Quality Mucus (and wet vaginal sensation)

CERVIX SYMBOLS: ● ● ○ ○ ○ ● ●

FERTILITY AWARENESS

Usual Time of Day

Month _____ Year _____ Cycle Number _____ Cycle Variation _____

Basal Body Temperature

99.0 —

98.0 —

97.0 —

Cycle Day	1	2	3	4	5	6	7	8	9	10	11	12	13	14	15	16	17	18	19	20	21	22	23	24	25	26	27	28	29	30	31	32	33	34	35	36	37	38	39
Date																																							
Day																																							
Intercourse																																							
Mucus																																							
Cervix																																							
Notes: Mucus Description:																																							
Sensation																																							
Disturbances, Schedule Changes, etc.																																							

MUCUS SYMBOLS:

✳ Menses

D
Dry
No Mucus
(and dry vaginal sensation)

M
Non-wet Quality
Mucus
(and dry vaginal sensation)

Ⓜ
Wet Quality
Mucus
(and wet vaginal sensation)

Ⓜ̶
Last day of
Wet Quality Mucus
(and wet vaginal sensation)

CERVIX SYMBOLS: ● ● ○ ◯ ◯ ○ ● ●

FERTILITY AWARENESS

Usual Time of Day _____

Month _____ Year _____ Cycle Number _____ Cycle Variation _____

Basal Body Temperature		
99.0	(rows 99, 9, 8, 7, 6, 5, 4, 3, 2, 1)	
98.0	(rows 98, 9, 8, 7, 6, 5, 4, 3, 2, 1)	
97.0	(rows 97, 9)	

Cycle Day	1	2	3	4	5	6	7	8	9	10	11	12	13	14	15	16	17	18	19	20	21	22	23	24	25	26	27	28	29	30	31	32	33	34	35	36	37	38	39	40
Date																																								
Day																																								
Intercourse																																								
Mucus																																								
Cervix																																								
Notes: Mucus Description:																																								
Sensation																																								
Disturbances, Schedule Changes, etc.																																								

MUCUS SYMBOLS:

✳	D	M	Ⓜ	⊗
Menses	Dry No Mucus (and dry vaginal sensation)	Non-wet Quality Mucus (and dry vaginal sensation)	Wet Quality Mucus (and wet vaginal sensation)	Last day of Wet Quality Mucus (and wet vaginal sensation)

CERVIX SYMBOLS: ● ● ○ ○ ○ ○ ●

FERTILITY AWARENESS

Usual
Time of
Day
_____ –

Month _____ Year _____ Cycle Number _____ Cycle Variation _____

Basal Body Temperature

99.0

98.0

97.0

Cycle Day	1	2	3	4	5	6	7	8	9	10	11	12	13	14	15	16	17	18	19	20	21	22	23	24	25	26	27	28	29	30	31	32	33	34	35	36	37	38	39	40
Date																																								
Day																																								
Intercourse																																								
Mucus																																								
Cervix																																								

Notes:
Mucus
Description:

Sensation

Disturbances,
Schedule
Changes, etc.

MUCUS SYMBOLS:

✳	D	M	Ⓜ	Ⓜ
Menses	Dry No Mucus (and dry vaginal sensation)	Non-wet Quality Mucus (and dry vaginal sensation)	Wet Quality Mucus (and wet vaginal sensation)	Last day of Wet Quality Mucus (and wet vaginal sensation)

CERVIX SYMBOLS: ● ● ○ ○ ○ ● ●

AFTERWORD

We hope that you've enjoyed *The Fertility Awareness Workbook* and through it have learned exciting, interesting and helpful information. After reading about fertility, some people find that they wish to have the information reinforced for them or the opportunity to share particular questions and concerns with someone knowledgeable about the information. If you find this is true for you, there are various ways to locate such a person. One way is through a fertility awareness class. Though there may not be such classes in all areas of the country, by contacting a church group, your state department of public health, or a family planning or local planned parenthood organization, you can learn what instructors and/or physicians are available to help you.

Since it is impossible for most people to "keep track" of the many new books related to fertility and sexuality being published today — much less read them all — we've listed a few that we thought might of interest to you.

BIBLIOGRAPHY
and List of References

Abraham, Guy E., M.D. *Pre-Menstrual Blues*. Opitmox, P.O. Box 7000-280, Palos Verdes Peninsula, CA 90274, 1981.

Anderson, Barry, M.D. and others. *The Menopause Book*. New York: Hawthorne Books Division of El Sevier, 1977.

Barbach, Lonnie Garfield, *For Yourself*. New Jersey: Signet Books, 1976.

Blandau, R. and K. Moghissi. *The Biology of the Cervix*. Chicago: University of Chicago Press, 1973.

Bartzen, Peter, M.D. "Effectiveness of the Temperature Rhythm System of Contraception," *Fertility and Sterility*. Birmingham: American Fertility Association, 1967.

Berkeley Holistic Health Center. *The Holistic Health Handbook*. Berkeley: And/Or Press, 1978.

Billings, E.L. "Symptoms and Hormonal Changes Accompanying Ovulation," *The Lancet*. London: Little Brown and Co., February, 1972.

Billings, Evelyn, M.D. *The Billings Methods*. Penguin, 1982.

Bing, Elizabeth. *Having a Baby Over 30*. New York: Bantam Books, 1978.

Borg, Susan and Judith Lasker. *When Pregnancy Fails*. New York: Beacon Press, 1981.

Boston Women's Health Book Collective. *Ourselves and Our Children*. Penguin, 1981.

Dalton, Katharina, M.D. *Once a Month*. Fontana, 1983.

Drake, Katia and Jonathan. *Natural Birth Control*. Thorsons, 1984.

Ferguson, Tom, M.D., ed. *Medical Self-Care: Access to Health Tools*. P.O. Box 717, Inverness, CA 94937: MSC, 1980.

Guay, Terry. *Your Personal Fertility Guide*. San Francisco: Harbor Publishing, 1980.

Hartman, Carl Gottfried. *Science and the Safe Period; a Compendium of Human Reproduction*. Baltimore: Williams and Wilkins, 1962.

Iffy, L., M.D. "Risks of Rhythm Method of Birth Control," *The Journal of Reproductive Medicine*. Chicago: Journal of Reproductive Medicine, Inc., September, 1970.

Julty, Sam. *Men's Bodies, Men's Selves*. [n.p.]: Delta, 1979.

Keefe, Edward F., M.D. "Self-Observation of the Cervix to Distinguish Days of Possible Fertility," *Bulletin of the Sloane Hospital for Women*. New York, 1962.

Kippley, J. *The Art of Natural Family Planning*. The Couple to Couple League, 1979.

Kippley, Sheila. *Breastfeeding and Natural Child Spacing*. New York: Penguin Books, 1977.

Luker, K. *Taking Chances: Abortion and the Decision Not to Contracept*. Berkeley: University of California Press, 1975.

Madaros, Lynda and Jane Patterson, M.D. *Woman Care*. New York: Avon, 1981.

Marshall, John. "Cervical Mucus and Basal Body Temperature Methods of Regulating Births-Field Trial," *The Lancet*. London: Little Brown and Co., August 7, 1976.

Mayle, Peter. *What's Happening to Me?* Macmillan, 1978.

Mayle, Peter. *Where Did I Come From?* Macmillan 1975.

Menning, Barbara Eck. *Infertility, A Guide for the Childless Couple*. New York: Prentice Hall, 1977.

Phillips, Angela and Jill Rakusen. *Our Bodies Ourselves: A Health Book by and for Women*. Penguin, 1978.

Phillips, Hazel and Tessa Hilton. *Girl or Boy? Your Chance to Choose*. Thorsons 1985.

Ratcliff, J.D. *Your Body and How It Works*. [n.p.]: Reader's Digest Press, Delacorte Press, 1975.

Reitz, Rosetta. *Menopause. A Positive Approach*. Allen and Unwin, 1977.

Ryder, Norman B. "Contraceptive Failure in the United States," *Family Planning Perspectives*, 5:133-142, 1973.

Seaman, Barbara. *Women and the Crisis in Sex Hormones*. New York: Bantam Books, 1978.

Shivanandan, Mary. *Natural Sex*. Hamlyn, 1979.

Stanway, Dr Andrew. *Why Us?* Thorsons 1984.

Vollman, R.F. *The Menstrual Cycle*. Major Problems in Obstetrics and Gynecology, v. 7 Philadelphia: Saunders, 1977.

A WORD ABOUT THE AUTHORS ...

Barbara Kass-Annese, R.N., B.S., N.P.

Barbara Kass-Annese is a leading instructor in Women's Health Care and Human Sexuality.

Consultant to the Department of Health & Human Services, she is a trainer in fertility awareness and Natural Family Planning for the southwestern and western states. Ms. Kass-Annese also serves as the project coordinator for the Los Angeles Regional Family Planning Council's Natural Family Planning Instructors' Training Program and conducts classes in human sexuality.

Born in Ohio, she earned her B.S. in Nursing and received her Nursing Diploma from Kent State University. After this she received Nurse Practitioner training through the Boston Family Planning Project and the University of California at Los Angeles — in Family Planning and Gynecology. This has been followed by educational programs at some of the leading hospitals throughout the United States — Harvard Medical School and New York University Medical School, among others.

Along with teaching Family Planning courses and writing several manuals for these programs, Ms. Kass-Annese often conducts seminars for colleges and hospitals.

Appearing often on radio and television, she covers a wide range of health care topics of interest to women and men, including family planning, human sexuality, fertility awareness, and Natural Family Planning.

Hal C. Danzer, M.D.

As a specialist in the field of reproductive health care, Dr. Hal Danzer is a reproductive endocrinologist in the Department of Obstetrics and Gynecology at Cedars-Sinai Medical Center in Los Angeles, California, where he also maintains a private practice, subspecializing in infertility and reproductive endocrinology.

Born in Montana, he moved with his family to southern California where he completed his education. Upon graduation from St. Louis University School of Medicine, he returned to Los Angeles to Intern at Los Angeles County — University of Southern California Medical Center. Following a residency in Obstetrics and Gynecology at Cedars-Sinai Medical Center, he completed a Fellowship in the field of Reproductive Endocrinology.

Active in both research and education, Dr. Danzer is an Adjunct Assistant Professor in Obstetrics and Gynecology at University of California at Los Angeles, Center for Health Services.

Serving as an investigator for one of the largest studies of Natural Family Planning, to date, he is also involved with ongoing clinical research in the area of Natural Family Planning.

INDEX